Color Atlas of Periodontology
Second edition

Color Atlas of
PERIODONTOLOGY

Second Edition

Ian M. Waite

PhD, BDS, FDS, RCS(Eng), FDS, RCS(Edin)
Head of the Department of Periodontology,
Vice Dean, Reader,
Consultant Dental Surgeon,
University College and Middlesex
School of Dentistry, London

J. Dermot Strahan

BDS, MGDS, RCS(Eng), FDS, RCS (Eng)
Head of Department of Periodontology,
Institute of Dental Surgery,
Consultant Dental Surgeon,
Eastman Dental Hospital, London

Clinical photography by:
Charles Day
Head of Photographic Department,
University College and Middlesex
School of Dentistry, London

James Morgan ARPS
Head of the Department of Medical Photography,
Institute of Dental Surgery,
London

Year Book Medical Publishers, Inc

Year Book Medical Publishers Inc.
200 North LaSalle Street
Chicago, Illinois
60601, USA

First published by Wolfe Medical Publications Ltd, 2-16
Torrington Place, London WC1E 7LT, UK.

ISBN 0-8151-8140-X

Library of Congress Cataloging-in-Publication Data

Waite, Ian M.
    Color atlas of periodontology/Ian M. Waite, J. Dermot Strahan. —
— 2nd ed.
        p.   cm.
    Includes bibliographical references.
    ISBN 0-8151-8140-X
    1. Periodontics — Atlases.   I. Strahan, J. Dermot. II. Title.
    [DNLM: 1. Periodontics — atlases. WU 17 W145cb]
RK361.W27 1990
617.6'32'00222—dc20
DNLM/DLC
for Library of Congress   89-70438
                                                                    CIP

CONTENTS

ACKNOWLEDGEMENTS

The authors wish to express great gratitude to the following for the contribution of photographs, slides and figures for the atlas, and for their very kind permission to reproduce this material:- The histological sections in Chapter 1 were from Berkovitz, B.K.B., Holland, G.R. & Moxham, B.J.: A Colour Atlas of Oral Anatomy (Wolfe Medical Publications Ltd). Histological and microbiological slides were contributed by Professors I.R.H. Kramer and H.N. Newman, Drs G.C. Blake, D.E.R. Cornick & A. Clarke and Messrs K.W. Lee, P.N. Galgut & M.B. Edwards. Acknowledgement is also due to the following authors of papers who kindly gave permission for diagrams to be reproduced from their publications: Professors M. Listgarten, H. Loe, H.R. Muhlemann & S.S. Socransky, and Drs J.C. Greene and A.D. Haffajee. These papers were originally published in the Helvetica Odontologica Acta, International Dental Journal, Journal of Clinical Periodontology, Journal of Periodontology, Journal of Periodontal Research, Oral Sciences Review, and an NIH Publication (USA). The authors are grateful to the editors of these publications for their cooperation.

Clinical and radiographic material has also been used from patients treated by various current or former colleagues at University College and Middlesex Dental School including Professors W.I.R. Davies, J.P. Moss, and R.N. Powell, Drs D.E.R. Cornick, A.T. Hyatt and G.J. Pearson and Messrs A. Edel, B.J. Groves & D.R. Wiley. Present and former colleagues at the Institute of Dental Surgery have also kindly contributed clinical photographs including Professor W.A.S. Alldritt, Messrs M.J. Shaw and V.J. Ward. Our acknowledgements and gratitude are extended to the above.

We wish to thank Mr Charles Day and Mr James Morgan for their time and skill in taking the clinical photographs.

In addition, we would wish to convey our thanks to the following who have helped with the typescript: Elizabeth Bagnall, Nancy Quesada and Alison Garvey.

One of the authors (J.D. Strahan) wishes to thank the other (I.M. Waite) for the time and skill displayed in the preparation of all the line drawings.

PREFACE

Over the past ten years there have been important changes in emphasis in periodontal theory and practice. The increase in scientific knowledge about periodontology has provided a firm basis for clinical treatment techniques. Treatment is more firmly based than ever on preventive concepts. Surgical techniques are used selectively, emphasis being placed on conservation of both soft and hard tissue. Periodontal treatment is being used increasingly in preparation for and as part of a combined treatment plan in both restorative and prosthetic dentistry.

The aim of this new edition is to present up-to-date theoretical concepts about periodontal disease and to relate these to current treatment procedures, to achieve an authoritative, contemporary review of the subject.

1 ANATOMY AND PHYSIOLOGY

The supporting tissues

1 Cross section of the tooth socket of a maxillary first premolar. The alveolar bone which provides support for the teeth is made up of the outer cortical plates, trabeculated cancellous bone and the bone of the sockets. Volkmann's canals perforate the sockets mainly in the coronal one third and carry blood vessels supplying the periodontal ligament. Anastomotic connections join these blood vessels to others entering the socket in the apical region and to those from the gingival margin.[1,2*]

*For references, see Bibliography, page 164.

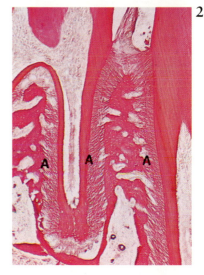

2 Longitudinal section of a mandibular molar tooth showing the oblique fibres (A) of the periodontal ligament. The teeth are attached to the sockets by bundles of connective tissue fibres comprising the periodontal ligament. Most of the fibres run apically in an oblique direction from bone to cementum. Near the crest of the alveolus and near the apex, however, the main orientation is perpendicular to the root surface. Illustration from Berkovitz, B.K.B., Holland, G.R. and Moxham, B.J. *A Colour Atlas of Oral Anatomy*, Wolfe Medical Publications Ltd.

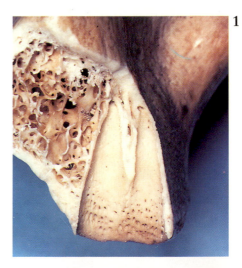

3 High power view of the periodontal ligament showing Sharpey's fibres inserted into bone (A) and cementum (B). The presence of numerous cementoblasts, fibroblasts and osteoblasts indicates a rapid rate of tissue turnover. The periodontal ligament also contains blood vessels, lymphatics, nerves and cell rests of Malassez. Special staining techniques can be used to enable a meshwork of fibres separate from the collagen bundles to be differentiated; these oxytalan fibres are probably associated with the vascular system.[3] Illustration from Berkovitz, B.K.B., Holland, G.R. and Moxham, B.J. *A Colour Atlas of Oral Anatomy*, Wolfe Medical Publications Ltd.

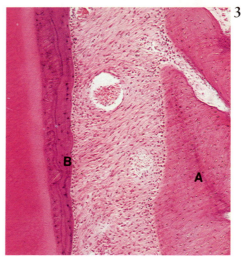

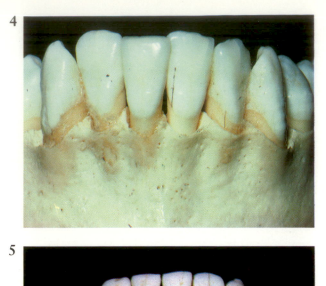

4 Marginal bone in mandibular incisor region. The crest of the alveolar bone socket in health is at a distance of 1-2 mm and follows the outline of the enamel-cement junction. The interproximal bone form depends on the contours of the enamel-cement junctions and on the proximity of neighbouring teeth; peak, plateau or shallow col formations are all commonly found.

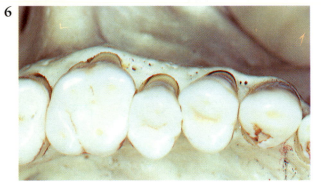

5 Marginal bone in mandibular incisor region demonstrating fenestrations and dehiscences. On the labial aspect of these teeth the circumscribed defects are fenestrations and the clefts are dehiscences. Regions most frequently involved by fenestrations and dehiscences are the facial aspects of canine teeth in both arches, mandibular incisor teeth and the palatal aspects of maxillary first molar teeth.[4,5] Where these defects exist they may predispose to gingival recession.[6]

6 Occlusal view maxillary posterior teeth. Teeth which are instanding in the arch are often associated with bony ledges, whereas those which are outstanding may have dehiscences and fenestrations.

The dento-gingival junction

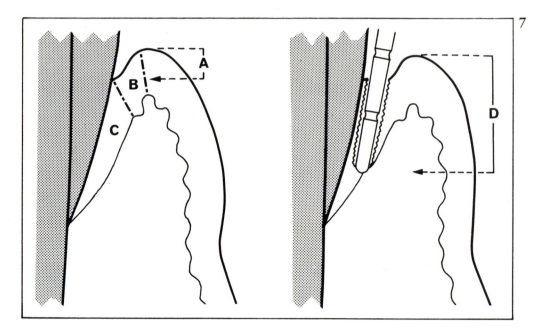

7

7 Gingival sulcus depths—contrast between anatomical and clinical. In health, there is a gingival sulcus (A) between the tooth and the gingiva which anatomically is about 0.5 mm in depth, and is lined by unkeratinised epithelium (B). At the base of the gingival sulcus the junctional epithelium (C) is attached to the tooth surface by hemidesmosomes via the basal lamina. Junctional epithelium is relatively weak and is disrupted to a varying extent by probing or other instrumentation. The clinical depth of the gingival sulcus (D) is thus greater than the anatomical depth of sulcus (A).[7,8,9]

8 Electron micrograph demonstrating attachment of junctional epithelium. The attachment of the junctional epithelium to the tooth is by hemidesmosomes (*white arrows*). Between the hemidesmosomes and the enamel (A) may be seen the basement lamina (B), comprising the lamina densa and the lamina lucida.[10] Illustration from Berkovitz, B.K.B., Holland, G.R. and Moxham, B.J. *A Colour Atlas of Oral Anatomy*, Wolfe Medical Publications Ltd.

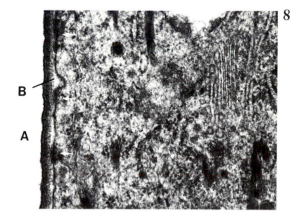

8

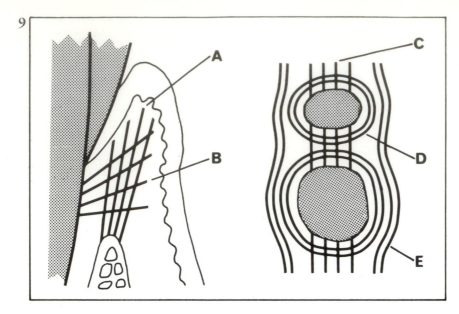

9 **Diagrams of connective tissue fibres of the free gingiva.** The collagen fibres of the gingiva contribute to the adaptation of the soft tissues to the tooth. They are classified as: (A) alveolo-gingival, (B) dento-gingival, (C) transeptal, (D) circular, (E) longitudinal. These fibre bundles mingle with each other.[11] The transeptal fibres may play an important role in maintaining the integrity of interdental contact points.

The investing soft tissues

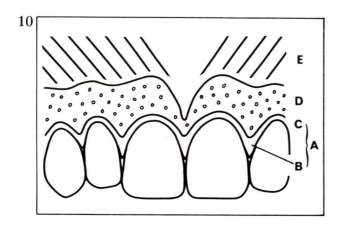

10 and 11 **Labial view of maxillary incisor region.** The free gingiva (A) is composed of the interdental papilla (B) and the marginal gingiva (C). A free gingival groove is present in some people and this corresponds approximately to the base of the gingival sulcus. The attached gingiva (D) extends from the level of the base of the gingival sulcus to the muco-gingival junction. The epithelium of the gingiva is keratinised or parakeratinised, and the corium contains dense collagen bundles which firmly attach the gingiva to bone and extra alveolar cementum. At the muco-gingival junction there is a change to non-keratinised alveolar mucosa (E). This is loosely attached to the periosteum and there are elastic fibres in the corium. The blood supply to the gingiva is derived mainly from the periosteal blood vessels. The interproximal papillae are supplied by capillary loops from the periodontal ligament and also from the crestal bone.[12,13]

12 Histological section of oral mucosa to show muco-gingival junction (Papanicolaou stain). It can be seen that the gingiva (A) is keratinised; there is a sudden transition to non-keratinised epithelium (B) at the muco-gingival junction (*arrow*). The stimulus for keratinisation has been shown to originate from the underlying corium; this effect is known as 'induction'.[14,15] Illustration from Berkovitz, B.K.B., Holland, G.R. and Moxham, B.J. *A Colour Atlas of Oral Anatomy*, Wolfe Medical Publications Ltd.

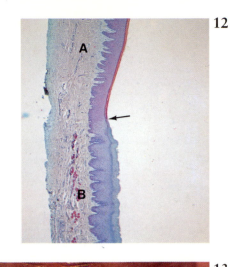

13 Naturally pigmented labial gingiva. The colour of gingiva and mucosa varies between individuals, ranging from pale pink to dark brown or black, the pigmentation being unevenly distributed.

14 Tapered gingival contour in maxillary incisor region. The convexity of the crown and the tapered margin of the free gingiva cause deflection of particles over the entrance of the gingival sulcus on to the outer keratinised surface of the gingiva.

15 Maxillary posterior occlusal view. The interproximal papilla is protected during mastication by the contact point and by the marginal ridges of the posterior teeth. Defective contact points may lead to food impaction with subsequent periodontal breakdown.[16]

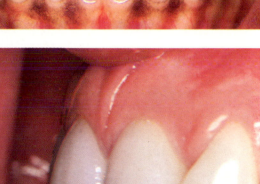

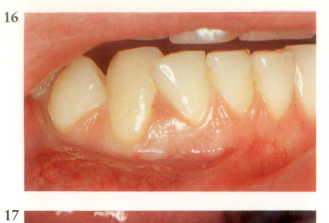

16 **Variations in the width of gingiva.** The width of the attached gingiva varies between individuals and also depends on the site in the mouth.[17] It has been suggested that a width of attached gingiva of at least 1mm is necessary for gingival health[18] but further studies have established that the width of attached gingival tissue neither influences the degree of inflammation nor the progression of periodontal disease.[19,20,21]

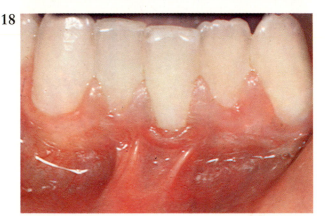

17 **Prominent mandibular lateral incisor with gingival recession.** It has been shown that prominent teeth are subject to dehiscences and, on these teeth, there may also be relatively thin gingival tissue. Trauma from heavy tooth-brushing pressure may contribute to recession, but it is necessary to instigate adequate oral hygiene measures, as reducing inflammation has been found to limit further recession.[22]

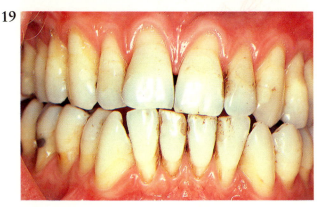

18 **High frenal attachment on labial aspect of mandibular incisor tooth.** A high frenal attachment may not only interfere with mechanical plaque control but may also result in there being no attached gingivae. There is consequent displacement of the gingival margin by muscle activity with the risk of plaque accumulation within the deepened sulcus. Combination of inflammation and muscle activity may lead to gingival recession.

19 **Acquired generalised gingival recession.** It has been suggested that a disproportion between the size of the alveolar processes and of the dental arches may predispose to bone dehiscences. The cause of generalised recession is often difficult to diagnose. Possible additional aetiological factors include chronic periodontal disease and trauma from incorrect tooth-brushing.[23]

Congenital and developmental abrnormalities

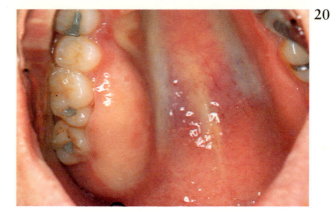

20   Enlarged maxillary tuberosities. Fibrous tuberosities are commonly associated with pocketing on the distal aspect of the last maxillary molar tooth and may extend anteriorly to the palatal aspects of the other maxillary molar teeth. These abnormalities frequently occur bilaterally.

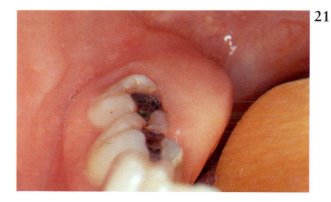

21   Mandibular retromolar enlargement. Similar enlargements are sometimes found in the mandibular retromolar region and also tend to be bilateral.

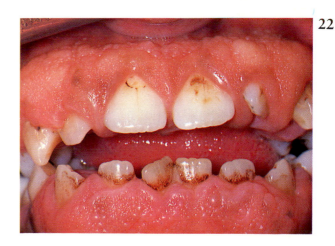

22   Fibromatosis gingivae. This is a relatively rare condition which may present with the eruption of the primary or secondary dentition or both. The aetiology is obscure and hence the condition has been termed idiopathic hyperplasia. A hereditary basis is supported by the occurrence of the lesion in blood relations.

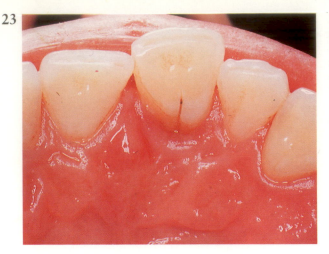

23

23 and 24   Palatal groove on maxillary central incisor tooth and radiograph of same tooth. Developmental abnormalities in tooth form may influence plaque retention and hence cause local exacerbation of periodontal disease. The groove on this tooth has allowed plaque to accumulate and spread up the root surface with resultant localised deep pocket formation. The radiograph shows an associated deep bone defect.[24,25]

24

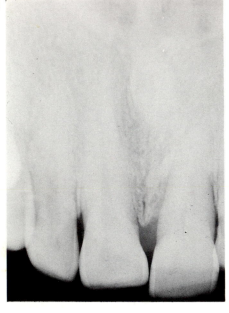

2 AETIOLOGY AND PATHOGENESIS OF PERIODONTAL DISEASES

Supra-gingival dental plaque

25 Bacterial plaque, early stage in formation (Gram stain). Supra-gingival plaque is formed by organisms in saliva adhering to the tooth surface or to an initial deposit of salivary pellicle. Supra-gingival plaque which has recently been deposited on a previously clean tooth surface comprises mainly Gram-positive cocci and rods.[1] Some of the micro-organisms associated with early plaque formation synthesise extra-cellular polysaccharides which enhance their adhesiveness, for example, *Streptococcus mutans* synthesises dextran.[2] The rate of bacterial colonisation is influenced by diet, dislodging forces, salivary factors and interbacterial feeding.[3]

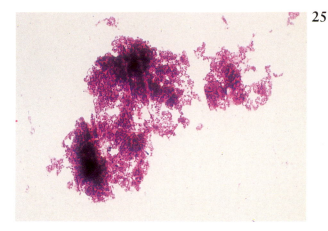

25

26 Bacterial plaque, later stage in formation (Gram-stain). As plaque accumulates there is a gradual increase in the proportion of Gram-negative cocci and rods, and of filamentous organisms and spirochaetes.[1] There is a decrease in oxidation-reduction potential as the layer of deposit becomes thicker. An increase has been found in *Actinomyces*, *Fusobacterium*, *Veillonella* and *Treponema* species in the later stages of plaque accumulation over a period of 3 weeks.[4] Some species of bacteria, for example *Streptococcus sanguis* and *S. uberis*, may inhibit pathogenic micro-organisms.[5]

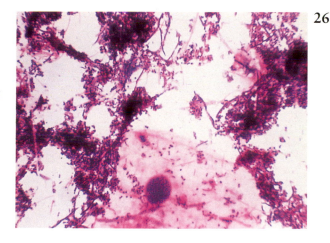

26

Gingivitis

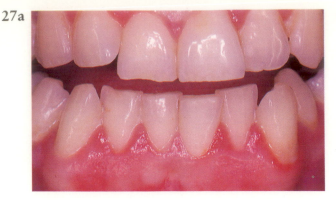

27a **Early gingivitis.** The relationship between dental plaque and gingivitis was verified in an experiment[6] in which all oral hygiene measures were withdrawn from a group of 12 subjects, comprising dental students or dental school personnel who, initially, had relatively healthy gingivae. During the study they each developed gingivitis within 10 to 21 days.

There are conflicting theories about the pathogenic mechanisms in the aetiology of gingivitis. Inflammation may occur as a result of an increase in the concentration of a broad range of bacteria (non-specific theory), or as a result of an increase in one or more particular species of *Streptococcus, Fusobacterium, Actinomyces, Veillonella, Treponema* or *Bacteroides* (specific theory). There is still controversy about which of these hypotheses is correct.[7,8,9,10]

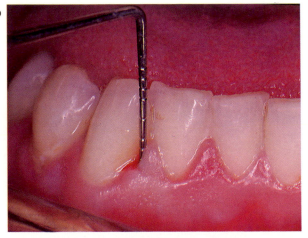

27b **The inflamed site.** The clinical signs of gingivitis include redness; swelling with resultant loss of tapered margins, interproximal grooves and stippling; bleeding on minimal trauma; exudate of gingival fluid. As gingivitis develops, there is a gradual opening up of the gingival sulcus resulting from the loss of connective tissue tone and the increase in turnover of junctional epithelial cells. A new ecological niche is thus formed which is relatively protected from the oral environment and which is continuously bathed in gingival fluid and products from local micro-organisms. The subsequent development of sub-gingival plaque species is strongly influenced by these environmental characteristics.[3]

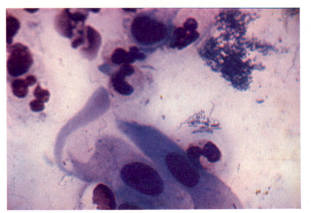

28 **Cells from the gingival sulcus.** A sample may be removed from the sulcus region on a plastic strip and stained as in this preparation. The largest cells are desquamated epithelial cells; there are various forms of bacteria present and in response to these there has been a migration of polymorphonuclear leukocytes.

The amount of gingival fluid increases as inflammation progresses. There are various constituents in this fluid, including lysozyme, metabolites from bacteria, leukocytes, immunoglobulins, complement and components, and various substances released from host cells including enzymes.[9]

Chronic adult periodontitis

29 Dark ground microscopy of plaque. The exacerbating factors in the progression of contained gingivitis to destructive periodontitis are not clear. The sub-gingival environment may favour an increase in periodontopathic micro-organisms, as a result of low oxygen tension, and the greater variety of nutrients. This environment favours the growth of Gram-positive rods such as *Actinomyces* species and the adherent plaque so formed may provide a basis for the subsequent attachment of a superficial layer comprising, for example, *Bacteroides* species or spirochaetes.[3]

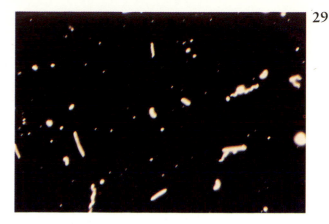

The types of micro-organisms in plaque have been assessed using phase contrast or dark ground microscopy. This technique has been used as an indirect method of determining periodontal disease activity at a site, but contradictory results have been obtained because only the morphology and motility of bacteria can be determined, not the species.[11,12] An additional factor influencing the progression to an active lesion may be an alteration in the host response.

More recent studies have investigated micro-organisms from active and inactive lesions of periodontitis, using relatively complex laboratory phenotyping techniques. At active sites, it was found that there were elevated levels of *Wolinella recta, Bacteroides intermedius, Fusobacterium nucleatum, Bacteroides gingivalis* and *Bacteroides forsythus*.[13,14]

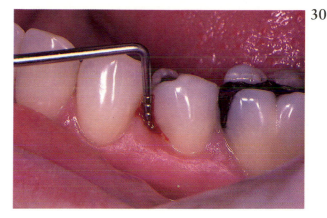

30 Periodontal pocket. At present there is no universally accepted clinical technique for detecting or predicting active periodontitis. The stability or rate of progression of loss of attachment may be determined retrospectively by comparing repeated assessment of pocket depth, measured relative to the enamel-cement junction.[15] To a varying degree there may be signs and symptoms of gingivitis, for example, bleeding on probing. In some cases, however, superficial inflammation may not be evident.

31 Radiograph of chronic adult periodontitis. Periodontitis may be recognised by radiographic assessment. In health, the bone level is about 2 mm apical to the enamel-cement junction, so an estimate can be made of any loss of interproximal bone. Serial radiographs may be used over a period of time to monitor the condition of periodontal bone. Marginal bone levels cannot usually be determined accurately from radiographs as they are obscured by the image of the tooth.[16]

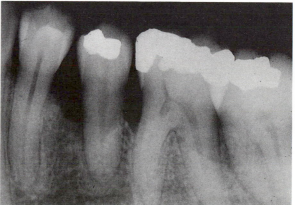

32

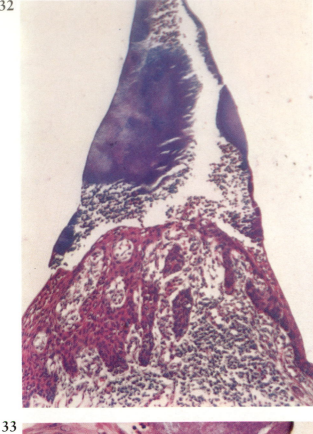

33

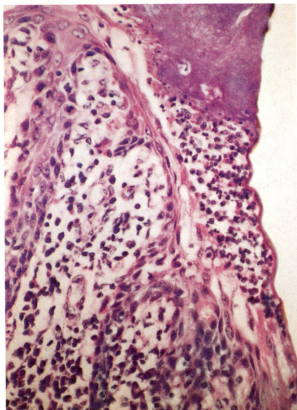

SUMMARY OF PATHOGENIC
REACTIONS IN GINGIVITIS AND
CHRONIC ADULT PERIODONTITIS

32 and 33   Chronic adult periodontitis (H & E
stained section) low power and high power view.
The pathogenesis of gingivitis and periodontitis is
complex. With the formation of sub-gingival
plaque, the micro-organisms are in direct contact
with the sulcular epithelium, which is unkeratinised
and only a few cells thick, enabling bacterial
products to penetrate into the subjacent connective
tissue.[17] Various bacterial products have been
implicated in the initiation and progression of
gingivitis and periodontitis; these include enzymes,
endotoxins, lipoteichoic acid, antigens and chemical
products, for example, ammonia and hydrogen
sulphide. The release of enzymes from plaque such
as hyaluronidase increases the permeability of the
epithelium and enables relatively larger molecules
to diffuse between the cells. An increase in oedema
and changes in the physical properties of the
connective tissue ground substance will aid
diffusion of irritants into the deeper tissues as the
inflammatory reaction develops.

Initially there is an acute inflammatory response
with a predominantly polymorphonuclear
leukocyte infiltrate. This gives way to a chronic
inflammatory response, typified by lymphocytes
and plasma cells which have been implicated in cell
mediated and antigen/antibody immune responses.
Although periodontitis with bone destruction may
be associated with chronic inflammation,[18] some
studies have shown that episodes of bone loss are
associated with localised acute inflammation, for
example, consequent to ulceration of the pocket
lining.[19]

There is controversy at present as to whether
there is bacterial invasion of the periodontal tissues
in periodontal diseases. Whereas several reports
have observed microcolonies of bacteria within
diseased tissue, the aetiological significance of these
findings is unclear.[5,20,21]

Stages in the development of the periodontal lesion

Four stages in the pathogenesis of chronic inflammatory periodontal disease have been described:[22] (A) the initial lesion, (B) the early lesion, (C) the established lesion, (D) the advanced lesion.

(A) THE INITIAL LESION

34   Blood vessel showing adherence of polymorphonuclear leukocytes prior to emigration into the connective tissue—electron micrograph (EM). Within 2 to 4 days of the accumulation of bacterial plaque, there is an acute inflammatory reaction in the connective tissue immediately adjacent to the junctional epithelium. Polymorphonuclear leukocytes adhere to the inner walls of the blood vessels and, in response to chemotactic factors, migrate between the endothelial cell junctions. The vessel walls become more permeable to fluid with resultant oedema in the surrounding tissues.

35   Polymorphonuclear leukocyte migrating through junctional epithelium (EM). There is increased migration of polymorphonuclear leukocytes via the junctional epithelium into the gingival sulcus. The leukocytes insinuate a passage between the epithelial cells and, in the later stages of inflammation, may disrupt the continuity of the epithelial barrier.

(B) THE EARLY LESION

36   Lymphocytes and a plasma cell in connective tissue (EM). The vascular changes and the accumulation of leukocytes are more pronounced than in the initial lesion, and by about 4 to 7 days there is an increased number of lymphocytes in the locally affected connective tissue adjacent to the junctional epithelium. These intermediate-sized lymphocytes may undergo transformation into sensitised T- and B-lymphocytes and plasma cells. There is a continuing decrease in the collagen content of the infiltrated connective tissue. Some of the changes of the early lesion may be associated with a cellular immune response involving T-lymphocytes and lymphokines. There is continuing migration of leukocytes through the junctional epithelium. The basal cells of the epithelium begin to proliferate and there is rete peg formation.[23]

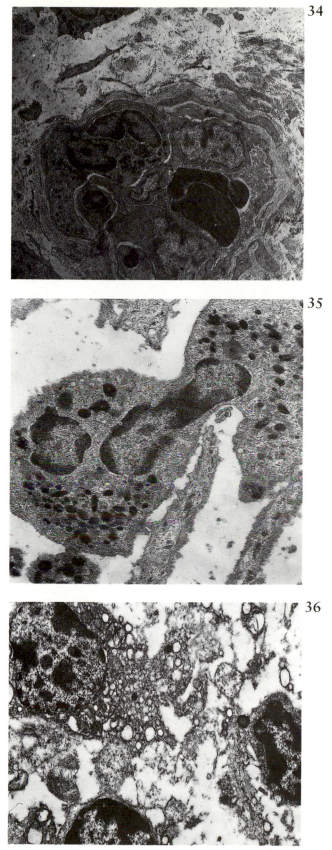

34

35

36

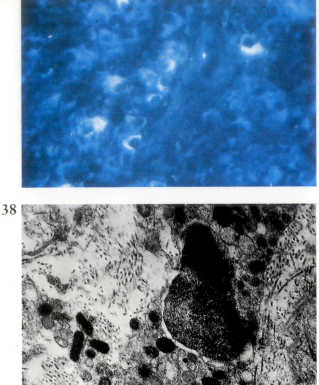

(C) THE ESTABLISHED LESION

37 Plasma cell containing immunoglobulins, demonstrated by immunofluorescence. The cellular infiltrate adjacent to the connective tissue now contains predominantly plasma cells. These cells are also found along blood vessels and between collagen bundles deeper within the connective tissue. The chronic inflammatory reactions in the established lesion may be mediated by antigen/antibody reactions. The junctional and sulcular epithelium may proliferate and migrate into the infiltrated connective tissue and along the root surface, thus being converted to pocket epithelium.[23,18] The detachment of junctional epithelium and its conversion into pocket epithelium enables further downgrowth of plaque.

38 Polymorphonuclear leukocyte with granules being released (EM). The continuing migration of polymorphonuclear leukocytes is brought about by chemotactic factors in plaque and also by antigen/antibody reaction. The release of lysosomes from polymorphonuclear leukocytes during phagocytosis of foreign material, or on their death, may enhance local tissue damage.

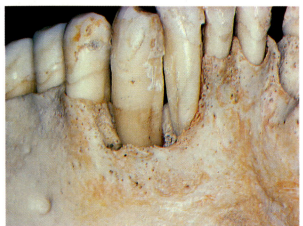

(D) THE ADVANCED LESION

39 Bone loss in periodontitis. The advanced lesion in the pathogenesis of periodontitis is typified by resorption of bone which occurs episodically. During active phases, epithelial ulceration has been noted and it has been suggested that the associated acute inflammation may be a cause of the bone destruction. The aetiology is not certain, however, and is probably caused by a change in balance between bone formation and bone resorption, as a result of a combination of factors; action of various bacterial products, for example, endotoxin and lipoteichoic acid; release of lymphokines, such as osteoclast activating factor from T- and B-lymphocytes; release of active factors, for example, prostaglandins from macrophages and polymorphonuclear leukocytes.[18,19,24,25]

Plaque retaining agents

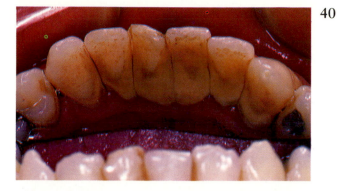

40   Supra-gingival calculus. A number of factors can enhance plaque retention and hence contribute to the progression of periodontal diseases. Supra-gingival calculus is formed by deposition on to the tooth surface of calcium, phosphate and other ions from saliva. This calcified deposit is white or cream and is most commonly found near the openings of the ducts of the submandibular and parotid salivary glands. There are several theories about calculus formation:[26]

(a) Calcium and phosphate ions in saliva are in a supersaturated solution and, hence, are liable to precipitate, especially where there are existing deposits to act as seeding agents.

(b) An increase in pH occurs with a greater tendency for precipitation as a result of the release of carbon dioxide when saliva enters the mouth; in addition, the rise in pH is enhanced by ammonia produced by plaque bacteria.

(c) An organic component of plaque may act as a seeding agent, causing the precipitation of inorganic salts within the plaque matrix.

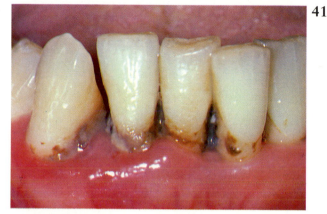

41   Subgingival calculus. Gingival recession has resulted in subgingival calculus becoming partly exposed. Subgingival calculus is dark brown or black. The deposits are usually found as localised thin layers in proximity to sites of soft tissue inflammation. These deposits are probably formed from substances in gingival fluid.[27] Both supragingival and subgingival calculus are attached to the tooth by mechanical interlocking in surface irregularities and, hence, are often very tenacious.

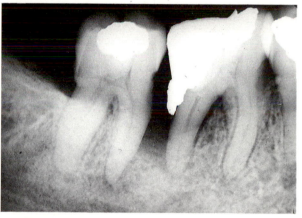

42   Defective margins of restorations. Ledges at the cervical margins of restorations encourage the accumulation of dental plaque and interfere with its removal. Where ledges are present, particularly if they are located sub-gingivally, there is a resultant increase in irritants and an associated exacerbation of gingivitis and periodontitis.[28,29] Studies emphasise the need to correct the contours of the margins of restorations as part of initial periodontal treatment (see **358** and **359**).

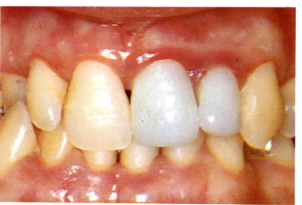

43   Defective crown margins. The porcelain jacket crowns on the left central and lateral incisors of this patient had marginal defects which could be detected by probing. The margins were located subgingivally and were inaccessible to cleaning procedures. As a result there was localised gingival inflammation (see **360**).

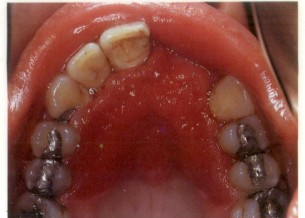

44 Palatal soft tissue beneath partial denture. Partial denture prostheses may also cause plaque retention with associated periodontal disease and inflammation of the denture bearing area. Investigation for infection by *Candida albicans* should be considered. This type of damage can be kept to a minimum, provided that good oral hygiene is maintained by the patient and that a satisfactory denture design is used.[30,31] Orthodontic appliances also increase plaque retention.

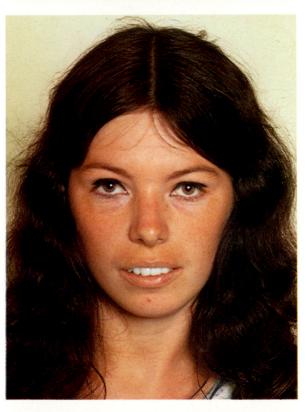

45 Incomplete lip seal. An incomplete lip seal will result in drying of the teeth and mucosal surfaces, and stasis of the salivary flow. The cleaning action of saliva and the removal of metabolites by diffusion will thus be interrupted.

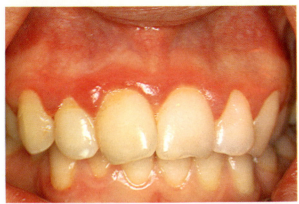

46 The gingival response. As a result of this interference with the cleansing and diluting effect of saliva, there will be an increase in concentration of the bacterial metabolic products in the plaque, with a localised increase in inflammation.[32]

47   Plaque and stain in a tobacco smoker. In a review of the effects of smoking on the gingiva, it was concluded that smoking worsened the oral hygiene status of the individual and that it acted as a co-factor with plaque, increasing gingivitis and periodontitis.[33] The defence of the host was reduced as a result of the depression of the chemotactic and phagocytic action of the oral polymorphonuclear leukocytes and there was a possible reduction in the immune response of the host with a lower level of circulating antibody. The effect of smoking on the blood supply to the gingiva is controversial; a recent study has suggested that it may be increased.[34] There is very strong evidence that smokers are more susceptible to acute necrotising ulcerative gingivitis.

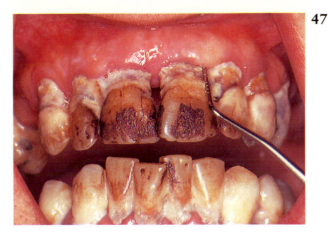

3 PERIODONTAL DISEASES OF EARLY ONSET, AND REFRACTORY DISEASES

In a number of relatively rare periodontal conditions there is an exaggerated rate of periodontal bone loss. For some of these conditions, laboratory investigations have revealed associated systemic abnormalities but the effect of these minor systemic factors on the general health, in most cases, is minimal.[1]

Prepubertal periodontitis

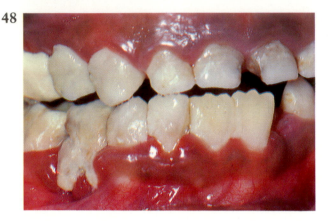

48

48   Prepubertal periodontitis—localised form. This may affect the primary dentition of children from about 4 years old onwards.[2] There are localised and generalised forms of the disease (see Papillon Lefevre syndrome, **64** to **66**). In the localised form, functional defects have been found in either the polymorphonuclear leukocytes or monocytes, whereas in the generalised form both types of cell may be affected. In the generalised form otitis media, skin and respiratory tract infections are common. Recommended treatment is by plaque control and thorough root planing, with systemic antibiotic as an adjunct, although clearly at this age tetracyclines should be avoided in order to prevent intrinsic tooth staining. The response to treatment depends on the severity of the involvement and is very poor in the generalised form of the disease. Subsequently, the permanent dentition may be involved.

Juvenile periodontitis

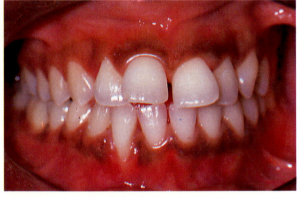

49

49 and **50**   **Juvenile periodontitis (periodontosis), clinical and radiographic features.** This is a relatively uncommon disease of uncertain aetiology. The clinical presentation has been described thus:[3]
(a) It affects adolescents and teenage children from 11 years old onwards.
(b) There is often a hereditary background.
(c) No obvious, direct correlation can be seen between local aetiological factors and the presence of deep periodontal pockets.
(d) There is a very distinctive radiographic pattern of alveolar bone loss, the one side being a mirror image of the other.
(e) The rate of progression is relatively rapid.
(f) There is no involvement of the primary teeth.
(g) According to most reports, a greater number of females than males are affected.

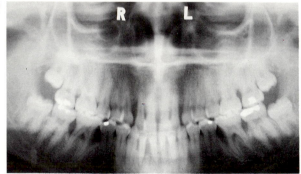

50

51 Radiograph of younger sister of patient shown in 49 and 50—greater bone loss. Studies into the genetics of juvenile periodontitis have indicated that it may be inherited either as an autosomal recessive disease or as an X-linked dominant disease.[4] It is more common in A and B blood groups than in O.[5] No linkage between the juvenile periodontitis gene and HLA antigens has been found.[6]

The exact prevalence figures for juvenile periodontitis are difficult to assess as some of the studies inappropriately included adults, but prevalence ranges from 0.1 per cent in European subjects to about 5 per cent in Indian, Middle Eastern and Afro-Caribbean subjects.[7,8,9]

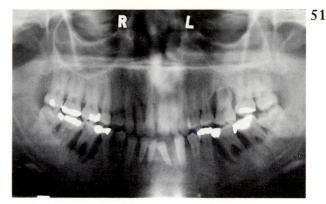

51

52 Radiograph of generalised juvenile periodontitis. This form is more common in females and in older patients; it is probable that the disease begins as the localised form and in some subjects progresses to become more generalised.[10,11]

Recent research has established that there are various changes in leukocyte function in patients with juvenile periodontitis, including reduced neutrophil chemotaxis which may be modulated by both serum and bacterial factors. These changes have been seen in some, but not all, types of juvenile periodontitis.[12,13,14]

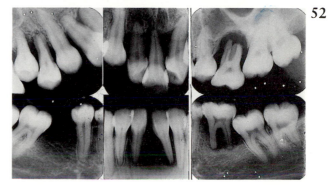

52

53 Juvenile periodontitis—same patient as in 52. Usually only very thin layers of plaque are found on teeth affected by juvenile periodontitis. Various micro-organisms have been implicated in the aetiology of the disease.[15] One which has received considerable attention recently is *Actinobacillus actinomycetemcomitans* (a non-motile, Gram-negative, coccobacillus). Increases in this micro-organism have been found in almost all studies of patients with localised juvenile periodontitis, with an associated elevation in antibody levels to *A. actinomycetemcomitans* in serum, saliva and gingival fluid. Another micro-organism that may be involved is *Capnocytophaga gingivalis*.[16] Micro-organisms have been found invading the gingival connective tissues in localised forms of juvenile periodontitis. Several pathogenic products are produced by *A. actinomycetemcomitans*, including capsular polysaccharides which aid adherence to mucosal surfaces, leukotoxin which inhibits leukocyte chemotactic factors, and a substance which suppresses lymphocytes. Destructive factors produced by the organism include various toxins which can cause tissue damage and bone resorption, a number of different enzymes including phosphatase and collagenase, and an epitheliotoxin.[17,18,19]

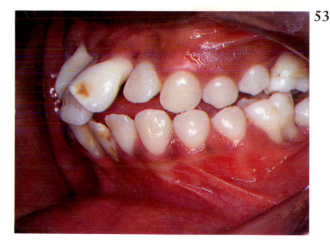

53

54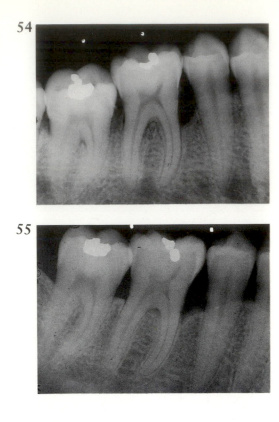

55

54 and **55** **Treatment of juvenile periodontitis—pre-operative film showing bone defect on lower right first molar teeth and radiograph taken 2 years after periodontal surgery showing reduction of bone defect.** Treatment is based upon plaque control to a meticulous standard.[20] Often it is necessary to use periodontal surgery to treat residual soft tissue pockets and bone defects. This patient was treated by curettage of all granulation tissue from osseous defects with conservation of the bony walls. Other techniques that have been used include osseous surgery, induced eruption, autogenous iliac marrow graft and tooth transplantation.[21]

In view of reports describing micro-organisms within the gingival tissue, the use of antibiotic treatment, for example tetracycline, has been recommended in addition to conventional therapy.[22,23] It has been suggested that tetracycline should be administered in 250 mg doses, 4 times per day and that this regime should be continued for at least 2 to 3 weeks.[24] The results of surgical treatment without antibiotic therapy have been found by some workers to be less good than the combined regime.[25] Following all treatment methods, careful long-term maintenance is essential.[26]

56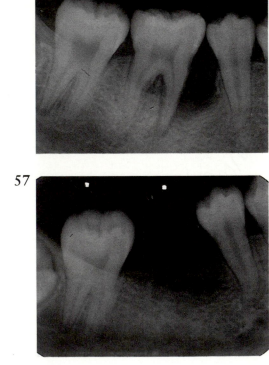

57

56 and **57** **Mandibular first molar region and same region one year after extraction.** Where bone loss is severe in juvenile periodontitis, selective extraction may be the most satisfactory treatment. As can be seen, healing of the socket resulted in elimination of the bony defect. The prognosis of the neighbouring teeth was greatly improved by loss of the severely involved first molar tooth. Having established a stable condition around the abutment teeth, prosthetic replacement can then be planned as necessary.

Rapidly progressive periodontitis

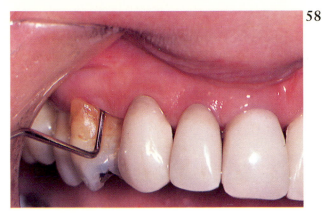
58

58   A 28-year-old patient with rapidly progressive periodontitis (quiescent phase). Rapidly progressive periodontitis occurs in young adults of 20 to 35 years of age.[2] During the active phase the gingivae are extremely inflamed with proliferation, haemorrhage and exudation. There may be temporary malaise, weight loss and depression. Most patients have serum antibodies for *Bacteroides gingivalis* or *Actinobacillus actinomycetemcomitans* or both. There are defects in either neutrophil or monocyte chemotaxis, and motility studies of the neutrophils show an enhanced random migration.[4,27]

59 and 60   Radiographs of patient in 58, at presentation and showing change in bone level over 12 months. There is rapid destruction of alveolar bone over a period of a few weeks or months. The disease may progress without remission to tooth loss or, alternatively, it may become quiescent. Patients may respond favourably to meticulous plaque control treatment with root planing or periodontal surgery, especially when this is accompanied by antibiotic therapy as described in 55; a proportion of patients, however, respond less satisfactorily to treatment.[2]

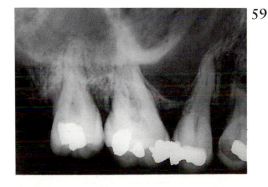
59

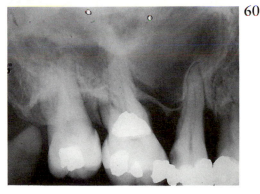
60

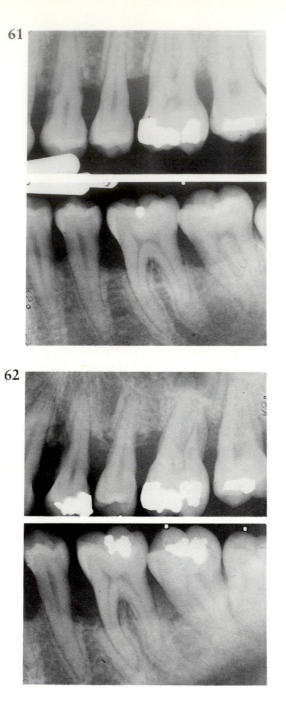

61

62

Refractory forms of periodontitis

61 and 62 Radiographs of left posterior teeth of a 53-year-old female, at presentation and showing changes over 2 years. This patient underwent a course of periodontal treatment which included plaque control, root planing and periodontal flap surgery. In spite of good co-operation by the patient and regular visits for professional maintenance of plaque control, there has been continuing bone loss. Several studies have documented that about 10 to 20 per cent of patients treated for advanced periodontitis suffer from continuing loss of attachment and bone destruction after treatment.[28,29,30] *Actinobacillus actinomycetemcomitans* and *Bacteroides gingivalis* have been detected at sites where disease was progressing. These refractory forms of periodontitis require more frequent maintenance appointments; periodic treatment with antibiotics, as described in 55, may be beneficial if there is evidence of recurrent inflammation.[31,32]

4 SYSTEMIC FACTORS INFLUENCING HOST RESPONSE

The microbial composition of plaque and the response of the periodontal tissues to it varies as a result of local factors, and under the influence of inflammatory and immunological reactions. In addition, a number of specific systemic factors have been shown to influence the response of the host and may be classified thus: congenital and developmental; hormonal changes and diseases; blood dyscrasias; nutritional disorders; drugs.

Congenital and developmental

DOWN'S SYNDROME

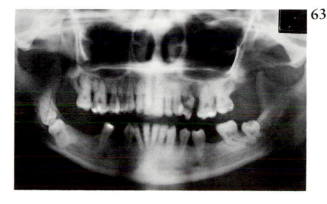

63 Radiograph of 18-year-old girl with Down's syndrome. In patients with Down's syndrome, from childhood onwards there is an increase in gingivitis and periodontal destruction when compared with subjects having similar social conditions and comparable levels of plaque.[1,2] A relatively frequent incidence of previous episodes of acute ulcerative gingivitis has been reported.[3] The cause of these changes has been linked with several factors, including abnormalities of both tooth anatomy and periodontal connective tissue, reduced T-cell function and functional defects of PMN leukocytes and monocytes.[4]

In the management of these patients, the need for frequent visits for oral hygiene instruction has been stressed and the use of electric tooth-brushes, fluoride pastes and chlorhexidine mouthwashes is recommended.[5]

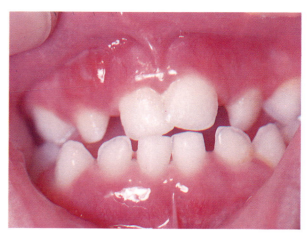

64 Papillon Lefevre syndrome. This is a rare disorder probably inherited as an autosomal recessive trait with parental consanguinity being observed in many cases.[6] Histologically, the gingival lesions are dominated by plasma cells, although it has been reported that the immunological status of the patient is normal with no disorder in lymphocyte transformation test or polymorphonuclear leukocyte function.[7,8,9]

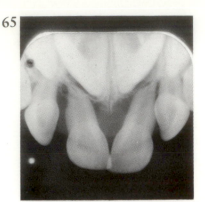

65 Radiograph of maxillary incisors (same patient as in 64). Both the primary and secondary dentition are affected by a rapidly destructive periodontitis necessitating tooth extraction within a few years of eruption.[10,6]

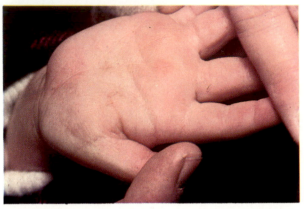

66 Palm of hand (same patient as in 64). The other characteristic feature of the syndrome is that the epidermis of the palms of the hands and soles of the feet is thickened and feels rough as a result of hyperkeratosis.

Hormonal changes and diseases

PUBERTY GINGIVITIS

67 Gingival condition in puberty. During puberty there may be an increase in gingivitis; the changes in host response to plaque are thought to be caused by altered hormonal levels. Children with established chronic gingivitis on entering puberty tend to be more severely affected.[11]

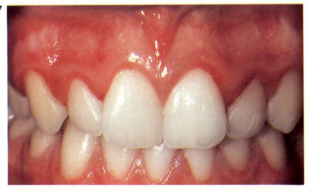

68 Clinical response 10 days after oral hygiene instruction. The establishment of effective plaque control resulted in resolution of the gingivitis, thus demonstrating that the disease is primarily plaque-associated and the hormonal effects are a secondary factor.

PREGNANCY GINGIVITIS

69   Gingival condition at 6 months. The hormonal changes during pregnancy also cause an enhanced host response to plaque.[12,13] As with puberty, healthy tissues tend to be unaffected and changes occur only where plaque and gingivitis are present initially.[14] The changes are probably caused by a raised level of progesterone which results in increased permeability of blood vessels and changes in ground substance. The plasma levels of oestrogen during pregnancy show a close correlation to the levels of *Bacteroides melaninogenicus* in subgingival plaque, and this can be attributed to the metabolic requirements of these micro-organisms.[15] It has been reported that oral contraceptives may result in similar but less severe changes to those in pregnancy.[16]

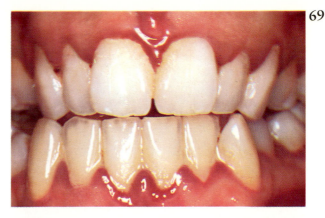

70   Same patient as in 69 after parturition. After parturition, gingival inflammation more or less resolved to the level present before pregnancy and there was no loss of attachment.[13] Treatment of periodontal disease during pregnancy generally should be restricted to scaling, root planing and improved oral hygiene. Any decision regarding the need for periodontal surgery should be left until hormonal levels have returned to normal.

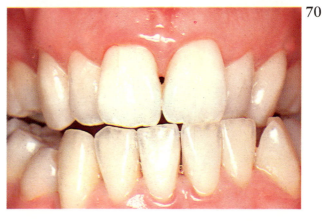

MENOPAUSE

71   Desquamative gingivitis. Following the menopause there may be changes in the epidermis, including thinning of the epithelium and a tendency to desquamative change. Recent reports suggest that with modern laboratory tests some of these desquamative lesions may be diagnosed as dermatological disorders such as lichen planus, benign mucous membrane pemphigoid, pemphigus or psoriasis.[17] The influence of hormone replacement therapy on these conditions remains unexplored.

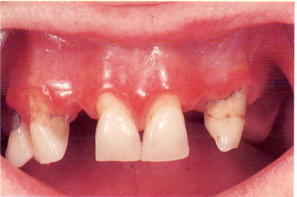

DIABETES MELLITUS

72   Clinical condition of 40-year-old diabetic. This condition may be associated with severe gingivitis and periodontal breakdown. It has been demonstrated that diabetic patients have more inflammation and loss of attachment than non-diabetic patients; some studies have reported increased bone loss especially in patients with long-standing diabetes.[18,19] The changes may be related to neutrophil chemotaxis[20] and capillary fragility caused by changes in the basement membrane.[21]

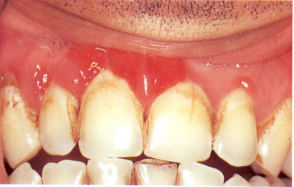

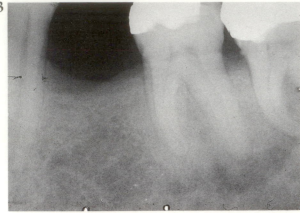

HYPERPARATHYROIDISM

73 Radiograph in hyperparathyroidism. This shows the ground glass appearance of the bone in hyperparathyroidism. The appearance of localised gingival enlargements (see **105** and **106**) should be followed by excision and biopsy, as the histological appearance of giant cells in conjunction with ground glass or osteoporotic lesions of the bone make checking of serum calcium and phosphorus levels essential. This condition may also be associated with renal stones.

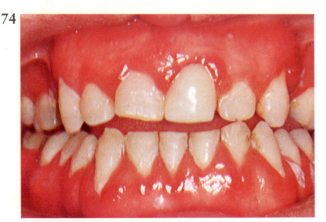

Blood dyscrasias

74 Agranulocytosis may induce gingival changes. A number of blood dyscrasias including agranulocytosis and cyclic neutropaenia may produce marked changes in the gingival tissues caused by alteration in the number and function of leukocytes. Ulceration of the mucosa and abscess formation are also common.

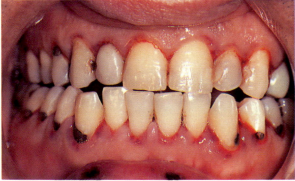

75 Acute monocytic leukaemia in a 45-year-old male during the early stages of anti-leukaemic therapy. The presence of leukaemia may first be diagnosed as a result of oral changes which include spontaneous bleeding and oedematous gingival enlargement; there may also be bruising and ulceration of all mucosal surfaces. The markedly improved results of current medical treatment make the long-term management of many patients with leukaemia practical. In general, periodontal management involves maintaining plaque at a low level and removing plaque-retentive factors. The dentist should be aware that as a result of the active phase of therapy and the associated systemic changes there may also be mucosal lesions.[22,23]

Nutritional disorders

Changes in the periodontal tissues associated with an inadequate diet tend to be found rarely and only in the socially deprived or in those with unusual and inadequate dietary habits. Examples may be seen in elderly people, alcoholics and drug addicts. Periodontal changes associated with nutritional inadequacies of a general nature, such as in kwashiorkor have been reported in tropical areas.[24]

76   Vitamin C deficiency may result in gingival changes. In its most severe form this condition affects the connective tissues of the periodontium. The clinical changes of severe gingivitis and mobile teeth are accompanied by more general problems. If a nutritional cause is suspected, the level of ascorbic acid can be tested and appropriate doses prescribed.

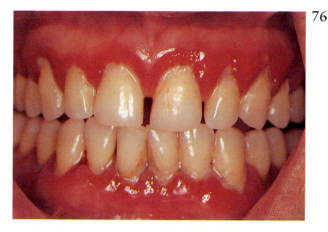

76

Drugs

77   Gingival hyperplasia associated with hydantoin. Patients taking hydantoin drugs for epilepsy may develop gross fibrous proliferation of the soft tissue in response to plaque, with resultant gingival pocketing. This effect becomes self-perpetuating as consequent increased retention of plaque in these pockets exacerbates the inflammation and hyperplasia. It is thought that these changes may also be associated with changes in calcium metabolism. Good oral hygiene and removal of deposits have been shown to reduce the proliferation of tissue but surgical excision of the hyperplastic tissue often proves necessary, for aesthetic or functional reasons. Patients should be warned, however, that hyperplasia may gradually recur, necessitating further localised surgery.[25]

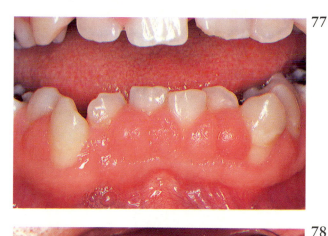

77

78   Gingival reaction to nifedipine. This anti-anginal drug is effective against both vasospastic and exertional angina. Nifedipine also has the ability to alter calcium metabolism[26] and acid mucopolysaccharide metabolism.[27] In patients taking this drug, gingival hyperplasia has been reported which clinically and histologically resembles that caused by hydantoin. The gingival condition should be treated in the same manner as hydantoin hyperplasia.

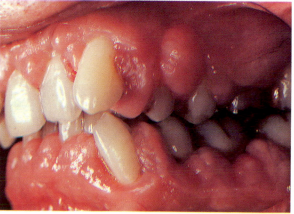

78

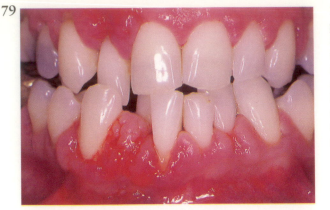

79 **Cyclosporin has altered tissue response to plaque.** Cyclosporin, an immuno-suppressive drug, is used in association with organ transplants, and in the treatment of type I diabetes mellitus and other auto-immune conditions.[28] Histological specimens show a picture closely resembling hydantoin hyperplasia. The gingival changes may prove very difficult to control by removal of irritants and surgical treatment may be contraindicated by the medical condition.[29]

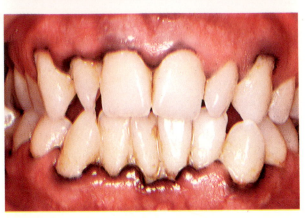

80 **Pigmentation of gingiva caused by systemic bismuth.** Drugs or pollutants can cause acquired gingival pigmentation. This illustration, taken some years ago, shows discoloration of the gingivae caused by bismuth therapy. The systemic ingestion of other metals or metallic compounds, for example mercury, lead, arsenic or silver, can also cause gingival pigmentation. The discoloration is enhanced in the presence of marginal inflammation and is probably caused by the precipitation of sulphide salts in the connective tissue.

SUMMARY

It may be seen from the above responses in the gingival tissues that a close examination is necessary so that any underlying systemic factors may be identified. In patients with these disorders, extra attention should be paid to preventive measures, in view of the enhanced response to plaque.

5 ACUTE PERIODONTAL CONDITIONS

Acute periodontal abscess

The inflammatory response comprises a range of reactions, with the acute phase at one extreme and the chronic phase at the other, the features of the responses tending to overlap in between. The type of inflammatory reaction is governed by the nature and intensity of the irritant and by the response of the tissues. The signs of acute inflammation are redness, pain, swelling, interference with function and raised temperature.

Acute types of periodontal disease are less common than chronic. The acute forms are generally caused by a proportional increase in the specific pathogenic micro-organisms, by a local predisposing cause, or by a change in the resistance of the host. It is important not only to diagnose the disease correctly, but also to ascertain the predisposing factor, as effective treatment should include elimination of the underlying cause, if possible. If the amount of inflammation seems to be exaggerated compared to the aetiological factors and if the response to treatment is slow, then the possibility of systemic disease interfering with the host response should be considered, for example, diabetes or a blood dyscrasia.

81 Periodontal abscess. A periodontal abscess is an acute purulent circumscribed infection, which occurs when there is an increase in the concentration or virulence of plaque micro-organisms. As a consequence, there is an ingress and build up of micro-organisms within the periodontal tissues around the pocket. The organisms implicated include Gram-negative anaerobic rods and Gram-positive organisms, such as streptococci and facultative or anaerobic rods.[1] *Actinobacillus actinomycetemcomitans* has also been implicated as a causative organism.[2] The symptoms may include pain on biting and swelling.

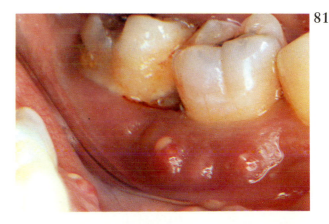

81

82 Radiograph of the same region as in 81. There are a number of factors predisposing to a periodontal abscess, for example deep pockets of complex morphology, infra-bony defects and multirooted teeth with furcation involvement. It has been suggested that an additional aetiological factor may be a constriction or blockage of the orifice to the pocket. Rapid bone destruction may occur locally as a result of the abscess.

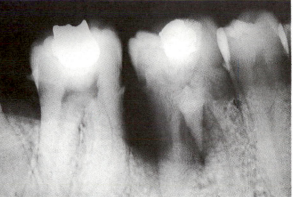

82

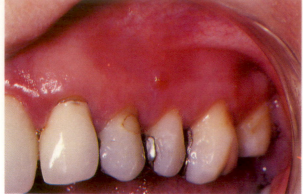

83

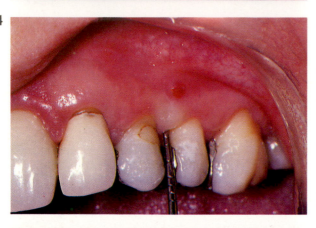

84

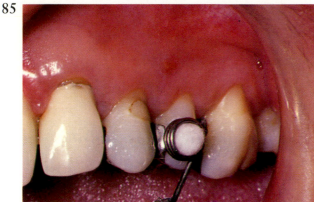

85

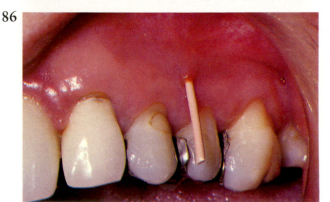

86

83   Clinical appearance and symptoms. The objective is to identify the cause of the sinus which is discharging on the buccal mucosa. A periodontal abscess and a periapical abscess may have a number of similar diagnostic features and differentiation between them must be based on a careful history and examination. The appropriate treatment can be planned only on the basis of a correct diagnosis.

Percussion tests may give an indication of which tooth is involved but will not differentiate between the types of abscess, as each may give rise to a positive response. When the abscess is draining, however, as in this case, percussion tests are often negative.

84   Periodontal probing. A fine probe should be used to detect periodontal breakdown. Circumferential probing is used so that even the narrowest of defects can be identified. It has been suggested that periodontal lesions are generally associated with relatively wide, conical-shaped pockets, whereas very narrow tract-like defects are usually caused by endodontic lesions discharging into the gingival sulcus.[3] In this patient, some pockets were found interproximally, the maximum depth of which was only 4 mm.

85   Vitality tests. The associated teeth should have their pulp vitality assessed by noting their responses to heat and cold and to electric pulp tests. In this case, the incisors and both premolar teeth did not respond to stimuli.

86   Probing the sinus tract. When present, a sinus tract can be probed either with a blunt instrument, for example a periodontal probe, or with a gutta percha point, as shown. The direction of the sinus tract may give an indication of the possible cause of the abscess—towards the apical region if endodontic in origin, or towards the cervical region if periodontal in origin.

87 Radiographic assessment. This will often help to confirm the diagnosis. The film was taken with the gutta percha point in the sinus tract, thereby enabling its direction and extension to be related to other radiographic features. The radiograph indicates that the first premolar tooth has incomplete endodontic treatment in one root canal and none in the other. The second premolar appears to have a periapical radiolucency and, as has been noted previously, did not respond to tests.

    The lesion was diagnosed as being periapical in origin, and the root canals of both the premolar teeth were cleaned and dressed before definitive endodontic treatment, the sinus tract subsequently resolving. The treatment of the co-existent early periodontitis, being a secondary factor, was managed conservatively.

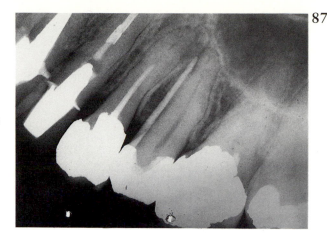

87

TREATMENT OF THE PERIODONTAL ABSCESS (see 244 to 246)

Acute phase

The acute phase is treated by root planing the involved teeth to the base of the pockets under local analgesia. Drainage of the abscess can be achieved usually by instrumentation within the pocket but, if the abscess is pointing externally and drainage after root planing has not been achieved, the abscess should be incised.

Antibiotics should be prescribed only if there is pyrexia or malaise, or extensive local spread of infection. Ideally, appropriate culture and sensitivity tests should be performed to determine the susceptibility of the causative organisms to the drug of choice.[4]

88 Periodontal abscess in the maxillary anterior region. This sinus between the left maxillary incisor and canine teeth had been present for several weeks and has not resolved after root planing, the patient still noticing a discharge from the area intermittently.

    The appropriate treatment should be decided after a complete assessment of the dentition. The advisability of extraction should always be considered as thereby excellent drainage is provided and, where bone loss is uneven, the loss of a severely involved tooth will often improve the prognosis of the neighbouring teeth (see 282 and 283). For this patient, the abscessed tooth is clearly an important one and further treatment would be carried out.

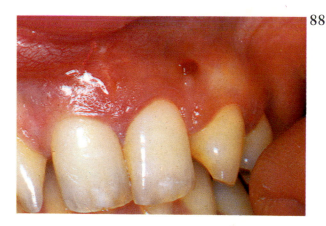

88

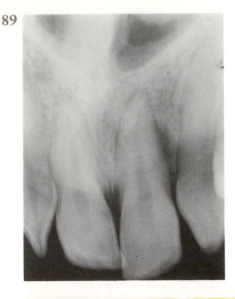

89 **Radiograph of anterior region.** The radiograph shows no evidence of a periapical lesion, and the anterior teeth gave positive results to pulp testing. There is bone rarefaction on the distal aspect of the central incisor tooth, indicating an infra-bony defect.

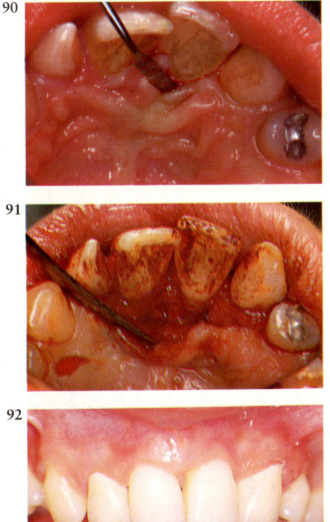

90 **Diagnosis of pocketing.** A pocket of over 6 mm was found on the palatal aspect. The associated periodontal abscess had tracked between the incisor and canine teeth to discharge on the labial aspect. After the acute phase, surgical treatment of an abscess is probably best undertaken without undue delay as there is a danger of recurrence. It has also been suggested that destruction as a result of acute inflammation has the best potential to heal, whereas if the lesion is allowed to become chronic there will be formation of a pocket with an epithelial lining and granulation tissue.[5,6]

91 **Surgical treatment.** An inverse bevel incision was used on both the palatal and labial aspects; the flap has been reflected and the granulation tissue removed by curettage. The bone defect associated with the abscess can be seen on the mesio-palatal aspect of the left central incisor tooth. Instrumentation at the base of the pocket was restricted to gentle debridement, with root planing further coronally. The aim of the procedure was to promote regeneration, so the emphasis was on conservative measures with restriction on the use of osseous surgery. Subsequently, the objective was to achieve good soft tissue adaptation and closure of the wound at the time of suturing.

92 **After treatment.** Six months after surgery the patient is symptom-free and the pockets have been eliminated. Several teeth have recently been crowned to improve aesthetics. The patient is now on long-term maintenance.

Acute necrotising ulcerative gingivitis (ANUG)

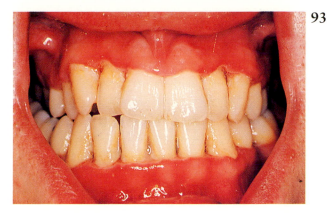
93

93 Clinical features. Acute necrotising ulcerative gingivitis is an increasingly rare acute inflammatory condition. Clinical features include ulceration and necrosis of the interproximal papillae, severe local pain and bleeding after minimal trauma. A common local factor is poor plaque control; contributory causes include calculus, partly erupted teeth, poorly contoured restorations and, additionally, tobacco smoking.[7] Physical or psychological stress may be supplementary aetiological agents, predisposing the individual to ANUG.[8,9] A depression of host defence mechanisms with reduced leukocyte response to chemotaxis and phagocytosis has been found.[10]

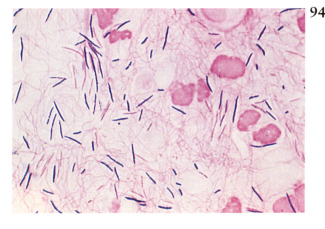
94

94 Micro-organisms from a patient with ANUG. This is a Gram-stained smear, showing numerous spirochaetes, fusiform bacteria and also epithelial cells. About 30 per cent of the microscopic count of ANUG plaque samples consist of various spirochaetal species (*Treponema*). The other bacteria seen generally include *Bacteroides intermedius* and *Fusobacterium* species.[8]

95 Treatment of the acute phase This is carried out by removal of the gross deposits, for example, by scaling with an ultrasonic instrument, in so far as the patient's symptoms of pain will permit. The invasion of micro-organisms into the periodontal tissues has been reported,[11] and the use of antimicrobial or antibiotic agents is probably indicated in many cases; for example, metronidazole or penicillin have been found to enhance the rate of resolution.[12]

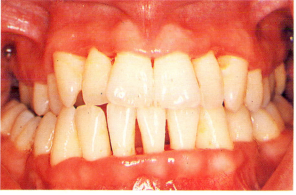
95

96 Results of protracted or repeated episodes of ANUG. The tissue destruction with ANUG can be very severe, as in this patient. In some areas of the world, in association with serious nutritional problems, ANUG has been found to progress more extensively to involve the buccal and labial mucosa and in a small proportion of cases to cause destruction of quite extensive areas of the face. Fortunately this condition, termed cancrum oris or noma, is very rare and is usually associated with a predisposing severe systemic infection.

The potential for relatively rapid destruction of the periodontal tissues in ANUG requires that every effort be made to obtain co-operation with plaque control and to stop tobacco smoking. The subsequent clinical treatment will include thorough root planing. If the patient maintains a good standard of oral hygiene, periodontal surgery may be of benefit to improve accessibility to clean, for example, where there are residual craters.

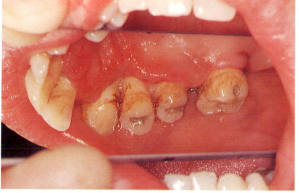
96

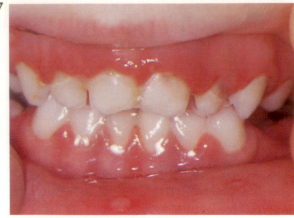

97

97 **Primary herpes simplex infection in a child.** Acute herpetic gingivo-stomatitis is caused by the herpes simplex virus, infection resulting in a disease of acute onset with pyrexia and malaise. The patient usually has a sore throat and there is a submandibular and upper cervical lymphadenopathy. The gingivae are swollen and bright red in colour. It is relatively unusual to find a vesicle that has not been ruptured by trauma.

98

98 **Mucosal lesions in a child.** The oral mucosa is often affected by vesicle formation, and lesions may be found on the tongue, palate, buccal mucosa and lips. The patient is treated, as for any viral infection, by rest; a soft diet with plenty of fluids is recommended. The pain and secondary infection of the oral lesions, which can be severe, may be helped by erythromycin elixir rinsed around the mouth after meals. After 12 years of age elixir of tetracycline may be used.

Dermal, genital, ocular or central nervous system involvement may occur. The last two are potentially serious as, respectively, blindness or death may result. Antiviral drugs, for example acyclovir, may be indicated for either topical or, in the case of more severe lesions, systemic use.

99

99 **Primary herpes simplex infection after resolution.** The lesions have resolved after 10 days, healing being the result of the production of antibodies to the virus. The change in antibody levels in the blood, from the initial presentation to the healed state, can be used as confirmation of the diagnosis.

100

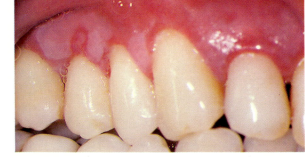

100 **Primary herpes simplex infection in an adult.** In the adult the ulcerated vesicles may be larger but fewer in number. The history of malaise and fever usually enables them to be distinguished from aphthous ulcers. Elixir of tetracycline may be rinsed around the mouth after meals. When treating any patient with active herpes infection it is even more important than usual that clinicians should wear rubber gloves, a mask and eye glasses, to protect themselves from infection.

101 Recurrent herpetic lesions. Recurrent herpetic lesions occur in approximately 30 per cent of the population. They are caused by latent virus being activated by local trauma or by systemic infections reducing the host resistance. They are common on the lip adjacent to the muco-cutaneous junction. Dental treatment is a common initiating cause. The topical application of an anti-viral agent, for example acyclovir ointment, may reduce the extent and duration of the lesions, provided treatment is started at the earliest signs.[13]

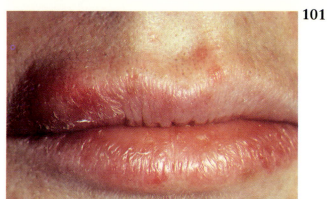

Gingival enlargement

Generalised gingival enlargement is commonly caused by plaque with resultant oedematous (see **140**) or fibrous enlargement (see **233**). Systemic factors may exaggerate the response; for example, hormonal factors (see **69** and **72**), drug therapy (see **77**), and blood dyscrasias (see **74** and **75**). In addition, generalised hyperplasia may be related to congenital abnormalities (see **22**).

Localised gingival enlargements also may have a variety of causes. Those related to developmental factors (see **20** and **21**) and acute localised infections (see **81**) are dealt with elsewhere. Other relatively common local enlargements are described below and it is important that a diagnosis be made to exclude the possibility of malignancy and other serious conditions.

102
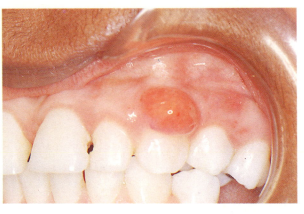

103
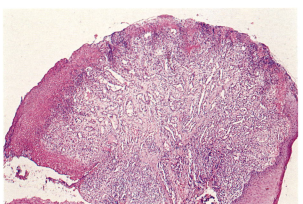

102 and **103** **Pyogenic granuloma—clinical and histological appearance.** The pyogenic granuloma arises in response to local irritation. It is often possible to detect calculus or a defective restoration associated with these enlargements. Treatment should be excision of the lesion, the tissue being sent for biopsy. On histological examination, the pyogenic granuloma is seen to be composed mainly of vascular tissue and fibroblasts. The surface epithelium is very thin and often ulcerated, in which case there may be an inflammatory infiltrate.

104 Pregnancy epulis—clinical appearance at 6 months. The pregnancy epulis, which is identical histologically to the pyogenic granuloma, may appear from the third month of pregnancy onwards and probably represents an intensified response to local minor trauma. Surgical excision is indicated during pregnancy only if the lesion is causing discomfort or interfering with eating. Removal after pregnancy is preferred as recurrence is probably less likely. The lesion is treated by excision and the underlying bone is curetted to ensure complete removal of affected tissue. All deposits must be removed from the teeth.

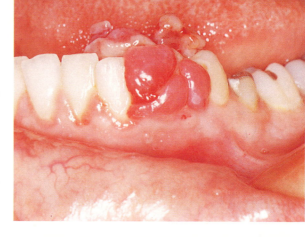

104

105 and 106 Peripheral giant cell granuloma—clinical and histological appearance. The peripheral giant cell granuloma may be found on the gingiva or the alveolar process and is often dark red or haemorrhagic. Histologically, it consists of a mass of reticular fibroblasts and multi-nucleated giant cells with numerous capillaries. There is usually no fibrous capsule. Treatment is by excision and curettage to include the base of the lesion. Recurrence is not uncommon, probably because there is no capsule.

The peripheral giant cell granuloma is similar in appearance to the giant cell lesions (brown tumours) of hyperparathyroidism and therefore radiographs should be taken to exclude a central lesion of bone. Patients with hyperparathyroidism may have renal stones and confirmatory tests include assessment of serum calcium, phosphorus and alkaline phosphatase levels (see **73**).

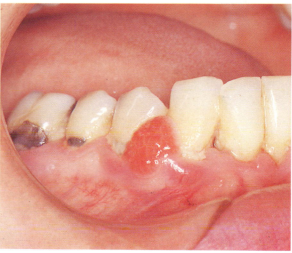

105

106

107 and 108 Fibrous epulis—clinical and histological appearance. The fibrous epulis, fibro-epithelial polyp and fibroma appear very similar clinically. The fibrous epulis, which is the most common of these, is a localised gingival swelling caused by chronic irritation and there are usually deposits of calculus on the associated teeth. Treatment is by excision down to bone, and biopsy. The fibro-epithelial polyp and fibroma may appear elsewhere in the mouth.

Histologically, the lesion is composed of fibrous tissue at various stages in development with blood vessels and inflammatory cells. There is a covering of well-differentiated stratified squamous epithelium.

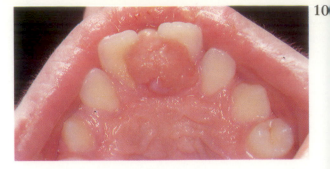

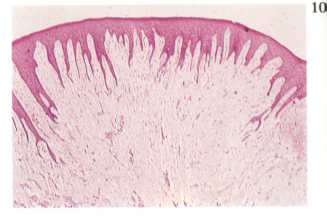

109 and 110 Papilloma—clinical and histological appearance. The papilloma is a relatively common lesion found on the tongue, lips, buccal mucosa, gingiva and palate. It is whitish in colour and may be pedunculated or sessile. Treatment is by excision to include the base of the lesion. Histologically, there are cores of thin connective tissue covered with epithelium which is hyperkeratinised.

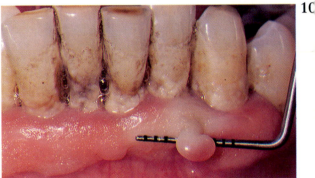

There are a number of uncommon benign and malignant neoplasms which may involve the periodontium but these are beyond the scope of this Atlas. Readers are referred to Tyldesley W.R., *A Colour Atlas of Oral Medicine*, Wolfe Medical Publications Ltd.

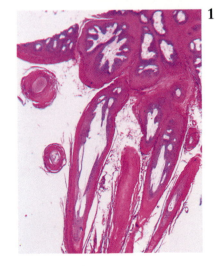

Mucosal lesions

There are several mucosal conditions which may occur either alone or in combination with other periodontal conditions. They may be of local origin or may reflect an underlying systemic condition. A correct diagnosis forms the basis of the subsequent treatment.

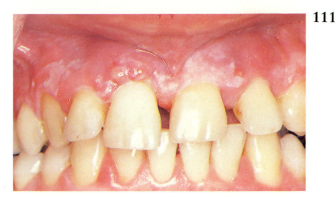

111   Chemical injury—ulceration of the labial gingiva and oral mucosa. Chemical injury to the gingiva and mucosa may result from the topical use of drugs. This patient has been using a mouthwash containing phenol. Another common cause of a localised lesion is an aspirin tablet retained in the mouth.

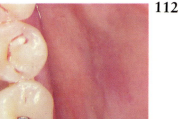

112   Physical injury—lesion in child caused by ballpoint pen. Habitual self-inflicted injury may pose a difficult diagnostic problem in children or adults because patients are frequently reluctant to admit to the habit. A biopsy may be necessary to exclude a systemic cause. The treatment should be directed towards helping the patient to recognise the cause and pointing out the long-term damaging effects. Psychiatric counselling should be considered for intractable cases.

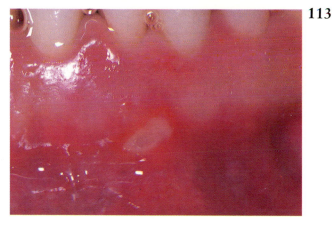

113   Aphthous ulcers. These occur singly or in groups and appear as painful, round or oval ulcers of varying size with an erythematous border. They may be found on the pharynx, tongue, palate, floor of the mouth, gingiva, cheeks or lips. They resolve after 1 or 2 weeks but there may be recurrence at varying time intervals. Many different forms of treatment have been recommended but none has universal application.

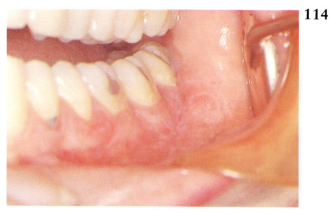

114   Lichen planus—clinical appearance of keratotic lesion. Lichen planus is one of the most common dermatological diseases to manifest in the oral cavity. The lesions are frequently bilateral and may occur on palate, tongue, floor of the mouth, gingiva, buccal mucosa and lips. Four types of lesion are described[1]: (a) papular keratotic, (b) vesiculo-bullous, (c) erosive, (d) atrophic. The different clinical presentations of the lesion complicate diagnosis, which should be confirmed by biopsy if there is any doubt. Biopsy of the erosive or atrophic varieties may be indicated because they may be pre-malignant conditions.

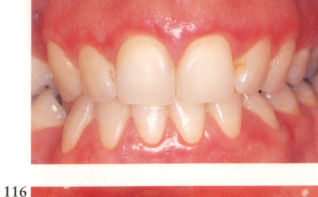

115 Desquamative gingivitis—erosive lichen planus. What used to be termed desquamative gingivitis can now usually be diagnosed more specifically, for example as erosive or atrophic lichen planus, benign mucous membrane pemphigoid, pemphigus or psoriasis. Correct treatment is dependent upon an accurate diagnosis based on clinical observation and on histological and immunological examination of biopsy specimens.[2,3]

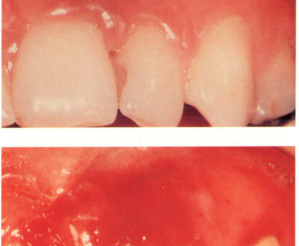

ACQUIRED IMMUNE DEFICIENCY SYNDROME (AIDS)

Infection by the human immune deficiency virus (HIV) has spread to all continents of the world during the past 10 years. In some cases the development of clinical AIDS may occur quite quickly but in others it may take many years, if ever, for symptoms to present. Oral lesions may include candidiasis, hairy leukoplakia, acute necrotising ulcerative gingivitis and Kaposi's sarcoma.

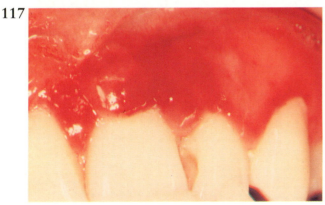

116 Early Kaposi's sarcoma in a male homosexual. This man presented with an unusual condition of the gingivae. Following counselling he was tested and found to be HIV positive and the lesion was diagnosed as Kaposi's sarcoma.

117 Kaposi's sarcoma—same case as 116, four months later. Despite scaling, root planing and oral hygiene instruction, the condition has deteriorated. Dental treatment for these patients is usually relatively conservative, the use of ultrasonic scalers being avoided to prevent aerosol infection.

118 HIV periodontitis. The clinical features shown are similar to those of acute necrotising ulcerative gingivitis with interdental cratering caused by loss of the papillae.

Epidemiology is the quantitative study of the occurrence and distribution of disease in groups of subjects. Scientific study of the epidemiology of periodontal diseases has been made possible by the development of appropriate indices. These comprise a series of definitions which enable the disease status of the periodontium to be measured and provide a method of quantifying the associated aetiological agents (see Appendix 3). Epidemiology may be used to measure the influence of such factors as age, sex, socio-economic status, race and geographic location on various periodontal diseases. The scope of the present chapter is the consideration of these aspects of epidemiology.

In addition, the assessment of aetiological agents, such as plaque and plaque-retaining agents and their influence on periodontal diseases, is also covered by epidemiology. This part of the subject, together with the influence of systemic disorders on the host response to bacteria is discussed in Chapters 2 and 4.

Influence of age and sex

PRE-SCHOOL CHILDREN

119   Gingiva of 5-year-old child. Apart from localised inflammation around erupting teeth, in the absence of systemic disease, gingivitis is generally not found in very young children. Thereafter, there is a steady increase in gingivitis. The reason for this increase may be an alteration with age in the response of the host, or qualitative changes in the plaque micro-organisms.[1,2]

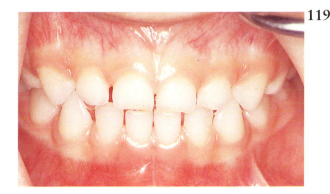

119

120   Graph showing relationship between gingivitis (PMA index) and age. In early teenage children there is a transient rise in gingivitis associated with the hormonal changes of puberty.[4,5] The hormone levels may influence the tissue responses to plaque by increasing the permeability of the soft tissues or modifying the inflammatory reaction. Alternatively, it has been suggested that the increased concentrations of sex hormones in gingival fluid favour the growth of some species of pathogenic bacteria, for example, *Bacteroides intermedius*.[6,7] After puberty, females tend to have less gingivitis than males, this trend continuing into adulthood.[8]

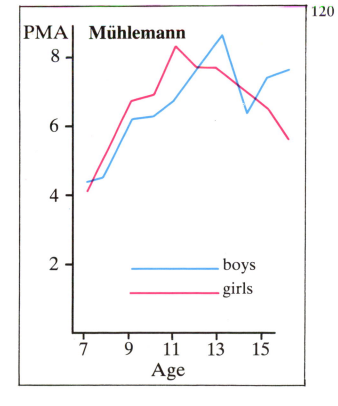

120

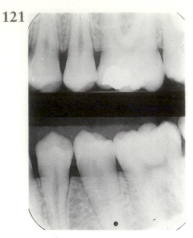

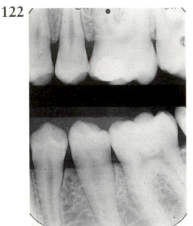

TEENAGE CHILDREN

121 and 122   Bite wing radiograph of 13-year-old child, and radiograph of same child at 15 years old showing minimal changes. There is disagreement about the incidence of periodontal destruction in teenage children; sociological factors probably have an influence. Where early bone changes have been diagnosed from radiographs, in both cross sectional and longitudinal studies, a wide range has been reported in the proportion of subjects in their mid-teens showing one or more sites with bone loss. The results range from 0.1 per cent to 51.5 per cent of individuals.[9,10,11,12,13]

Clinical measurements from the enamel-cement junction with a periodontal probe have detected loss of attachment of at least 1 mm at one site or more, affecting between 40 per cent and 96.5 per cent of 15-year-old children in north-west England. Those who had least education, and those of West Indian or Indo-Pakistani origin were more severely affected.[14] It is likely that a high proportion of these early, local changes can be attributed to gingival recession caused by trauma from brushing or mastication. The changes in bone may be caused by local tooth movement and responses to altered distribution of forces, as teeth erupt and take up their position in the arches. A review of periodontal diseases in children has been published.[15]

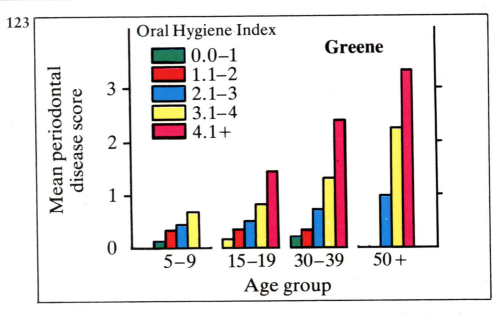

123   Progression of periodontal diseases (pooled results). Epidemiological studies have shown that during adult life there is a progressive increase in periodontal diseases with age. Where good standards of oral hygiene were maintained, however, the progression was minimal.[16,17,18] Thus, it was considered that an increase in periodontal destruction with age was caused by the prolonged exposure of the tissues to plaque metabolites with cumulative, incremental change.

50

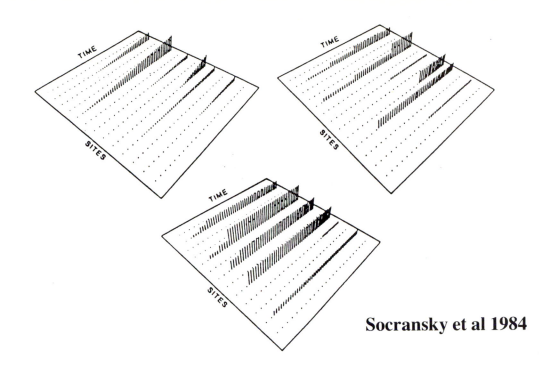

Socransky et al 1984

124   Diagrammatic representation of the progression of periodontal diseases. Epidemiological data based on average values may give a distorted representation of the natural history of periodontal diseases. Recent studies in individual subjects suggest that destruction may occur as the result of phases of irregular, episodic activity at individual or at multiple sites.[19,20,21] These suggestions are the subject of current debate.[22]

125 and 126   Radiograph of a patient with periodontitis, and same patient 2 months later with localised further destruction. Considerable variability in the susceptibility of patients to periodontitis has been reported. A relatively small proportion of subjects in any population group was found to be at greatest risk of suffering severe destruction.[23,24] Periodontitis is site specific and in 49 per cent of subjects destruction occurred only at localised sites. In 23 per cent of subjects there was more widespread disease and in 28 per cent generalised involvement was found.[20]

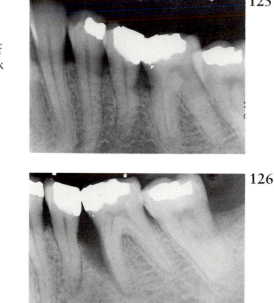

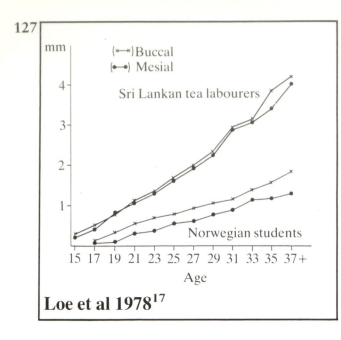

127

(×—×) Buccal
(•—•) Mesial

Sri Lankan tea labourers

Norwegian students

Age

Loe et al 1978[17]

Socio-economic factors, geographic distribution and effect of race

127 Londitudinal study of periodontal disease in Norway and Sri Lanka. This study compared subjects in developed and developing countries.[17] There is clearly a variety of factors that could account for the differences between the two groups including ethnic or nutritional factors. A major difference, however, was that the Norwegian subjects who had been on a preventive programme since school age had 60 to 70 per cent of all tooth surfaces free of plaque, whereas the Sri Lankan subjects who had never received any dental treatment or preventive care had plaque covering almost all tooth surfaces at each assessment. It was likely that other factors had relatively minor importance compared with plaque levels. The mean annual rate of loss of attachment for the Norwegians was up to 0.1 mm for the buccal and 0.05 mm for the mesial surfaces. For Sri Lankans these values were 0.2 mm and 0.3 mm respectively. It was probable that the cause of the relatively greater loss of attachment on buccal aspects for the Norwegians was trauma from brushing, whereas for the Sri Lankan group the greater loss was found interproximally and, thus, almost certainly was plaque-associated.

Developing countries

128 Periodontal support in 40-year-old subjects from Sri Lanka. The pattern of development of periodontal destruction was not regular in Sri Lankans; at 40 years of age the worst lesions were on the first molar teeth in both jaws and on the mandibular incisor teeth. At this age an average of 6 teeth had been lost from periodontitis; others were loose and severely affected.[17,25] Approximately 8 per cent of the population had a rapid rate of destruction with severely depleted dentitions by 40 years of age (less than 10 remaining teeth). Most subjects retained a complement of over 20 teeth well into their forties.[26]

Studies in Tanzania and South Africa have reported less periodontitis than in Sri Lanka in spite of abundant plaque deposits; for example, in Tanzania at 50 years of age an average of less than 1 tooth had been lost from periodontal causes.[24,27,28] It can be speculated that other factors besides plaque and age influence the rate of progression of periodontitis, as these subjects of African ethnic origin with very poor oral hygiene have a similar mean loss of attachment (2.2 mm total loss at 40 to 49 years of age) to those reported for Norwegian or American subjects.

128

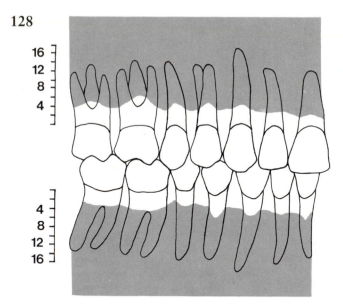

Loe et al 1978[17]

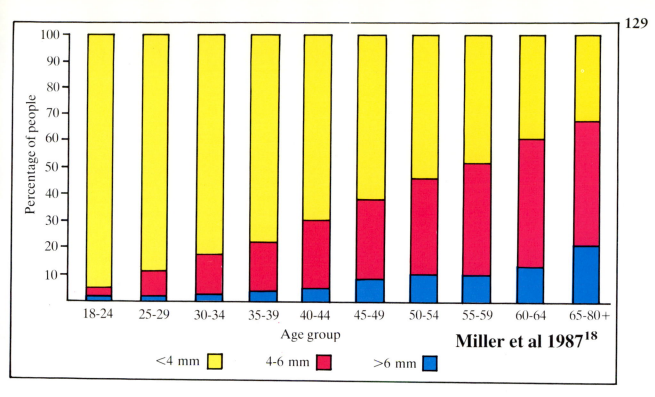

Developed countries

129 USA—percentage of people by most severe loss of attachment. The excellent condition reported in the previous study for the Norwegian subjects is supported by a recent extensive study in the USA in which they were found by 40 years of age to have a mean loss of attachment of only about 2 mm. By 60 years of age, the mean loss approached 3 mm. The American study reported that only a proportion of sites was involved, between 6 and 9 sites being affected on average, in the two age groups respectively.[18,29] In the same study it was reported that by 40 years of age, approximately 30 per cent of subjects had one or more sites with loss of attachment greater than 4 mm, and by 60 years of age this proportion had risen to about 60 per cent.

CLINICAL IMPLICATIONS

Periodontal diseases manifest in a variety of ways, with progression often being irregular and with different sites showing varying degrees of involvement. The susceptibility of individuals is not uniform. The rate of progression depends to a major extent on the quality of oral hygiene measures. In view of the variation in response to plaque between individuals, it is desirable to develop methods of predicting those at greatest risk, so that a waste of resources can be prevented. Intensive preventive measures will be necessary for those diagnosed as being at greatest risk.

Until prognostic indicators are available, ideally routine plaque control measures should be provided for everyone, with regular monitoring thereafter. At present, subjects at risk can be detected only retrospectively when the early signs of disease become evident. The necessary interceptive periodontal treatment should then be implemented without delay, followed by subsequent maintenance therapy.

It is essential that all dental patients are assessed at regular intervals for evidence of periodontal diseases. The various diagnostic criteria are discussed below.

A thorough case history provides the relevant background to the present dental condition of the patient, enabling the clinical picture to be related to any predisposing factors and to previous treatment. Taking a history, therefore, is fundamental to accurate diagnosis and will be used in planning subsequent treatment.

Medical history

A detailed medical history is essential, for the safety of operating personnel and the benefit of the patient. It enables a treatment plan to be developed which is compatible with the medical background. Many conditions will need confirmation by appropriate laboratory tests including haematological, chemical pathology, urinary assessments or biopsy. There are three major components:

1 Protection of operating personnel and other patients
In recent years the problems of cross-infection associated with Hepatitis B and AIDS have come to the fore and require special precautions.

2 Protection of the patient
Systemic conditions such as cardiac disease or bleeding diatheses may necessitate modification of the type and method of treatment. Recent or current drug therapy should be noted; also, any allergies to drugs which may be used in treatment.

3 Conditions influencing periodontal diseases
A number of medical conditions and drugs influence the response of the tissues to plaque and are therefore relevant to a correct diagnosis. They include pregnancy and diabetes, and drugs such as hydantoin and nifedipine. (See Chapter 4.)

Dental history

Presenting complaint
The patient is first asked about any general complaints, then about specific symptoms such as pain, swelling, bleeding, discharge or recession affecting the periodontal tissues. Chronic inflammatory periodontal disease, however, is often only associated with mild symptoms. In addition, it is important to enquire about mobility of teeth or their migration out of alignment in the arch.

History of complaint
Further information is sought about the date of onset of symptoms and about subsequent developments, including any recent treatment provided for the present condition, for example, drugs, scaling, root planing or periodontal surgery.

Oral history
A thorough knowledge of the previous oral history forms the basis of a comprehensive diagnosis. The patient is questioned about past dental treatment with detail of periodontal, preventive, restorative, prosthetic and orthodontic therapy. Habits such as tobacco smoking or betel nut chewing, which might affect the oral condition, are also recorded.

Oral hygiene methods
The patient is asked about any difficulty in cleaning the mouth or problems such as food impaction, also the frequency and method of tooth-brushing, the type of brush used and interproximal cleaning.

The examination
An extra-oral examination is carried out. Frequently, the case history may direct attention to a particular zone, for example, the temporo-mandibular joints or lymph nodes. The position of the lips at rest is also assessed (see **45** and **349**).

The intra-oral tissues are examined and all the mucosal surfaces in the mouth, including the pharynx, fauces, soft and hard palate, tongue, floor of the mouth, vestibule and buccal mucosa. A thorough oral examination of all patients is important, so that for example, if a malignant lesion were present it could be diagnosed and treated early. Mucosal lesions must be identified as, in some cases, the gingivae may be affected also; for example, lichen planus may be present on both the mucosa and gingiva (see **114** and **115**).

Attention is now turned specifically to the teeth and periodontal tissues. The attached and marginal gingivae and the papillae are assessed, and the distribution of gingivitis may be recorded on a chart (see **138**). Change in colour, consistency or contour and the presence of a frenum which encroaches on

to the attached gingiva is noted (see **18**). Where there is enhanced gingival response to plaque, specific tests are necessary to ascertain whether there is a systemic factor. Such tests may include haemoglobin concentration, differential white blood cell count, blood film for abnormal cells and blood glucose concentration (see **72, 74** and **75**).

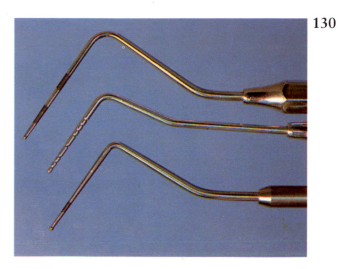

130

130 Periodontal probes. Several designs of periodontal probes are available (see also **30**). Operator preference will influence choice but generally the same type of probe should be used throughout treatment. Probing should be carried out on all aspects of the teeth. The initial emphasis is identification of pockets of 3 mm and over and, where such pockets are found, a general note should be made of their severity and distribution. Where deep pockets are present, especially where their distribution is uneven, complete periodontal charting is indicated.

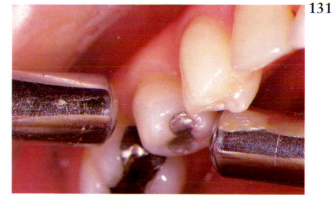

131

Mobility

131 and **132** **Detecting tooth mobility.** The Miller Index[1] is a commonly used clinical assessment in which instruments are placed on either side of the tooth and forces are applied bucco-lingually; mobility is scored 0 to 3. The system described here is a more sensitive modification of the Miller Index.[2] A score of 0 is where there is no detectable movement when force is applied. A score of 1 indicates barely distinguishable tooth movement. When the crown of the tooth moves up to 1 mm in any direction, mobility is scored as 2, and movement of more than 1 mm in any direction is scored as 3. Teeth that can be depressed or rotated in their sockets are also given a score of 3.

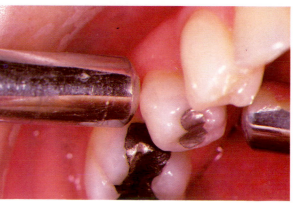

132

Tooth deposits

The amount and location of plaque deposits should be assessed. The plaque charts shown in Appendix 4 may be useful to record this information and, subsequently, they can be used to plan the patient's oral hygiene instruction. The distribution and quantity of supragingival and subgingival calculus is noted.

Occlusion

The Angle's classification is recorded. The occlusion is assessed with the mandible in the retruded contact position, in the intercuspal position, in lateral excursion and in protrusion. The articulation between these positions is checked and interferences noted. The patient is questioned about bruxism, clenching or other habits likely to exert excessive forces on the periodontium. If mobility is present it is correlated with these findings.

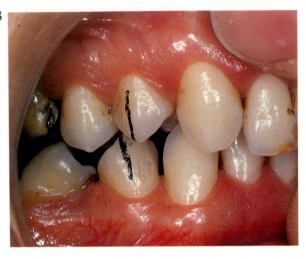

133

133 Determining retruded contact position—the vertical lines represent intercuspal position

Radiographic assessment

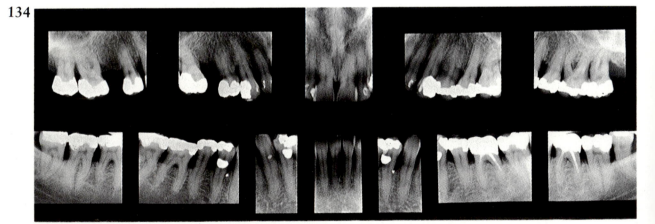

134

134 Periapical radiographs of patient using long cone paralleling technique. A variety of radiographic techniques may be used for detailed periodontal assessment. Periapical radiographs taken by long cone paralleling technique, as shown here, are ideal as they show the least distortion. A full mouth series comprises 14 films but for clarity only a restricted number is illustrated. These radiographs are from the same patient as in **135** and **138**. The upper right third molar tooth was extracted after the orthopantomograph had been taken, as it was causing pain from a periodontal abscess.

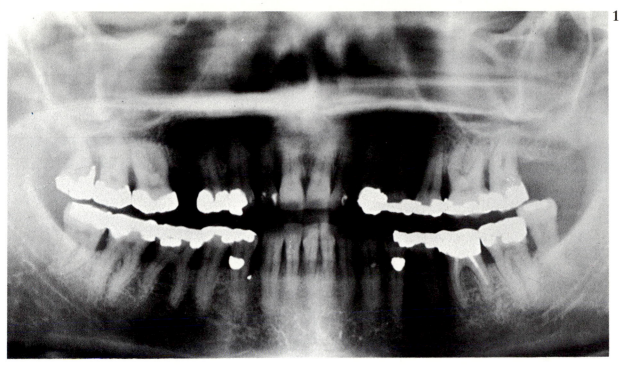

135 Orthopantomograph of same patient as shown in 134. Orthopantomographs provide a general view of the oral structures and a means of identifying relatively large pathological lesions or anomalies. They give an indication of the amount of periodontal bone destruction, but they are not suitable for accurate assessment of the degree of bone loss associated with individual teeth, as there is magnification and severe distortion and the outline of the bone margin is often not clear because of superimposition of extraneous intervening structures.

136 Vertical bite wing radiographs to show interproximal bone. Bite wing radiographs provide a good view of interproximal bone provided bone loss is not advanced. The vertical bite wing technique which, compared with the horizontal bite wing, involves rotation of the film through a right angle, provides an apical extension of the image.

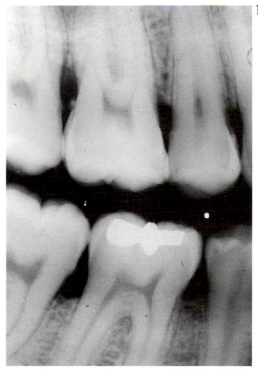

Assessment of periodontium

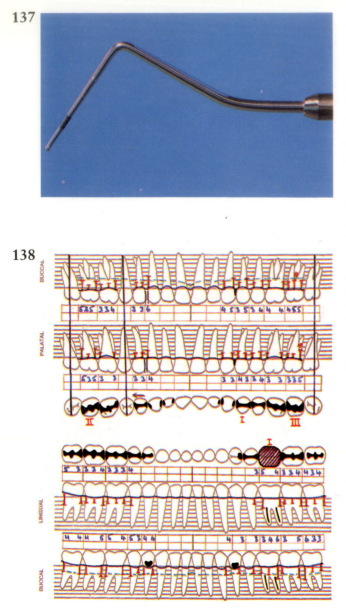

137 CPITN probe. One simple form of periodontal treatment planning that has been described may be carried out using the Community Periodontal Index of Treatment Needs (see Appendix 3). This involves probing the gingival tissues on 6 aspects of each tooth, using a special CPITN probe and recording the worst score for each segment. From this assessment it is possible to separate patients into those requiring relatively minor treatment and those who will require more extensive examination and treatment. Where pocketing is severe it will be necessary to complete a full periodontal chart.

138 Periodontal chart. There are various types of charts for recording the periodontal condition. Either a full periodontal chart can be compiled as illustrated or, for the less complicated case, this can be restricted to recording representative pocket depths in a simpler chart (see Appendix 4). The full chart is completed as follows: teeth which have been extracted are shaded in. Restorations and cavities are marked on the occlusal outline, and overhanging margins of restorations can be indicated on the lateral views. Any teeth which have had endodontic treatment are noted and a record is made of crowned teeth, pontics or removable prostheses.

The soft tissues are then assessed. The position of the gingival margin in relation to the enamel-cement junction is measured with a probe at the mesial, mid-marginal and distal sites on the buccal and lingual aspects of each tooth. The points are marked on the chart; each of the grid lines represents 2 mm. A blue line representing the gingival margin has been used to join these points.

The clinical depths of the pockets on probing are measured relative to the gingival margin at the same sites and recorded in the appropriate boxes. Where the depths exceed 2 mm, they are marked on the chart by a vertical red line. Asterisks are used to indicate furcation involvements.

When relevant, the position of the muco-gingival junction in relation to the gingival margin is measured and marked in with a broken line, which enables the position of the base of the pockets to be related to the muco-gingival junction. Frenal and high muscle attachments are outlined on the chart. The final procedure is to indicate irregularities in tooth position by arrows, for example over-eruption, drifting or rotation of teeth. Open contacts are represented by parallel lines. For comparison of changes after treatment, subsequent pocket depth recordings can be marked in the second row of boxes.

58

Summary—general treatment plan

The information obtained from the case history, clinical examination and radiological assessment is used to compile a treatment plan which must be designed to coordinate the various aspects of treatment (see Appendix 5).

Monitoring of the periodontal condition (Appendix 5)

The response to initial therapy, which necessitates seeing a patient over a period of several months to check healing, will be made much easier to assess if monitoring charts are used at each visit. An important indication of active inflammation may be the presence of bleeding on probing from periodontal pockets.[3,4] A useful way of recording the effectiveness of instruction and the patient's performance of oral hygiene measures may be to chart the presence or absence of dental plaque and inflammation at successive visits. Pocket depth measurements in relation to the enamel-cement junction should be repeated periodically.[5]

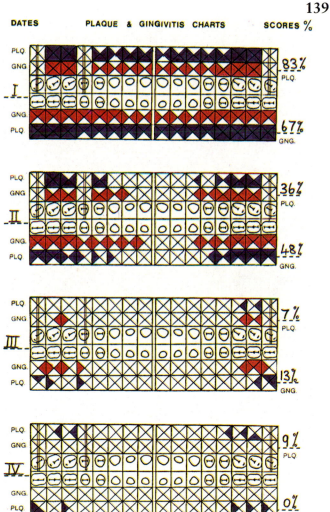

139 Charts illustrating changes in plaque and bleeding on probing, which took place over an 8 month period. Each triangular space on the chart represents 1 tooth surface; the presence of plaque on any surface is indicated as a shaded triangle on the chart. In the same way the presence of bleeding on probing is marked on the gingivitis chart. Percentage scores are calculated and may be used to encourage patients in the performance of their plaque control. In this patient there was a marked improvement over the first 4 months.

The control of dental plaque is the basis of both the prevention and treatment of periodontal disease. It is helpful if the patient's performance is monitored and there are several clinical parameters which can be recorded. Charts similar to those shown in **139** and Appendix 4 may be completed at intervals throughout treatment. The plaque and bleeding scores may be converted to percentages to give a general impression of the effect of treatment. These charts are of particular value in directing attention to problem sites.[1]

The objective of a plaque control programme is to establish a routine of a sufficiently high standard to result in the achievement and maintenance of a healthy mouth.

EDUCATION

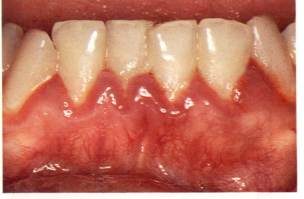

140   Patient with gingivitis. It is important that patients realise that they have a problem. This 22-year-old girl has marked chronic gingivitis with generalised deposits of plaque and calculus. She is informed in simple terms about plaque and the damage it does to teeth and periodontal tissues. The signs of disease are demonstrated in her mouth so that she can see and be encouraged by the subsequent improvement in the periodontal condition.

141   Disclosing agents. A disclosing agent is often useful in helping a patient to understand the distribution of plaque and its relation to gingivitis.[2]

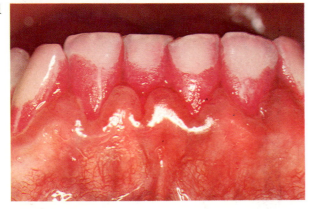

MOTIVATION

The first phase in effective treatment is to establish the patient's commitment to long-term retention of the teeth. It is essential that patients realise that the success of treatment depends at least as much on their own efforts as on those of the dentist. Motivation of the patient is based on the principles of encouraging success and reinforcing progress, rather than dwelling on negative aspects. The concept should be developed that oral hygiene is a part of routine daily grooming and self-care procedures, rather than a temporary treatment phase. Diligence on the patient's part will be rewarded by improved oral appearance and cleanliness and a reduction in the need for elaborate and costly periodontal and restorative treatment in the future.[3,4,5,6]

MECHANICAL PLAQUE CONTROL—ORAL AND FACIAL SURFACES

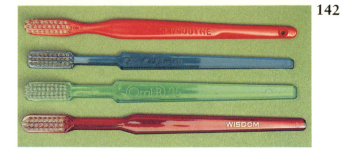

142 Conventional tooth-brushing. Clear information must be given on which type of tooth-brush is to be used and a sample should be provided to avoid confusion. A multi-tufted brush with a flat trim is suitable for most mouths and there are many examples available. The size and shape of the head and the design of the neck and handle should be considered so that the recommended brush provides access to all surfaces.

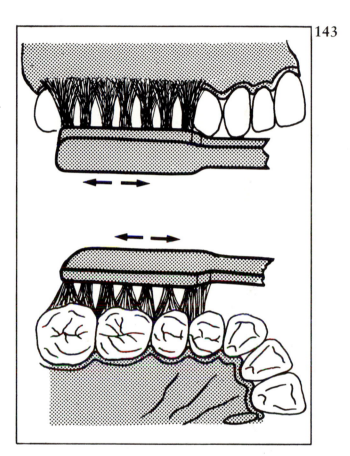

143 Tooth-brush technique. The Bass technique with various modifications has proved to be a very versatile procedure for removing plaque, even when arch form or gingival contour is not ideal. For the Bass method, the brush head is positioned at the dento-gingival junction with the filaments pointing into the gingival sulcus at 25° to the long axis of the teeth. The brush is then activated with a mesio-distal vibratory movement. There is a danger of causing mechanical trauma to the gingiva if the duration, frequency, direction or pressure of tooth-brushing is excessive or incorrect. Any such problems must be detected and corrected.[7]

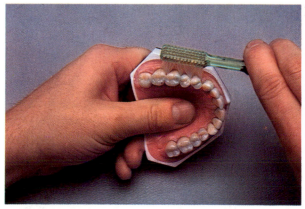

144 Demonstration models. Some patients find tooth-brushing technique easier to understand if it is first demonstrated on models. A systematic procedure for brushing must be established, each quadrant being cleaned in 3 sections, both facially and orally. The occlusal surfaces are then brushed.

145

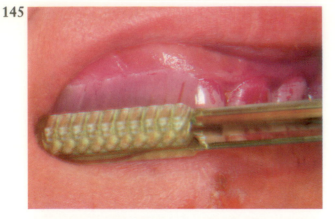

145 and 146   Instruction in the mouth and same patient attempting tooth-brushing. Tooth-brushing should be demonstrated in the patient's mouth, so that she becomes familiar with her own particular problems. In this way, she can recognise the correct action of the brush filaments on the gingiva by tactile sensation. The operator may choose to use one side of the mouth to demonstrate how disclosed plaque may be removed; the patient then attempts to repeat the procedure on the other side. Her hand may be guided by the instructor in the correct movements.

146

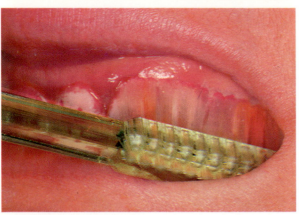

147

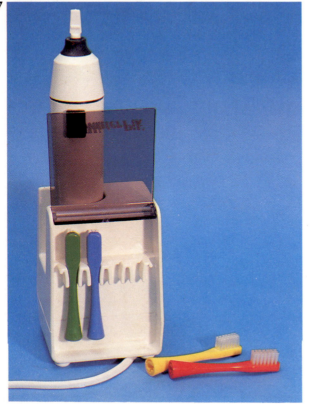

147   Electric tooth-brush. The electric tooth-brush may be useful for young or handicapped patients or for those with poor manual dexterity. Some patients prefer an electric tooth-brush to a manual one; both techniques appear to be equally effective.[8] The patient must be instructed to apply the filaments of the brush to the gingival margins and to follow a set sequence when using the electric brush.

148   Single-tufted brush. Some patients have difficulty in directing brushing activity towards the line angles and embrasure areas. A single-tufted tooth-brush may prove very useful in helping with this problem. It is also useful for cleaning irregularly aligned teeth and for teeth abutting a saddle area.[9,10]

1

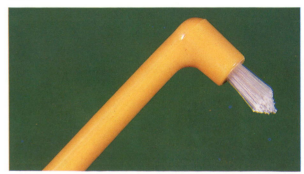

MECHANICAL PLAQUE CONTROL—INTERDENTAL SURFACES

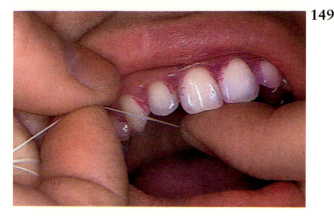

Interproximal cleaning may be carried out using dental floss, triangular wooden sticks or interdental brushes. Floss is ideal for small interdental spaces where there are convex or flat tooth surfaces. Waxed or unwaxed floss is available; some patients may find dental tape easier to hold. These various possibilities have been found to be equally effective.[11]

Wood sticks require less manual dexterity than floss and are quicker and more convenient to use, but they are not as effective at cleaning lingually or sub-gingivally.[12] Where there are concavities in the surfaces of the teeth or soft tissue interproximally, interdental brushes may be used provided there is sufficient space for the brush head (see **156**).

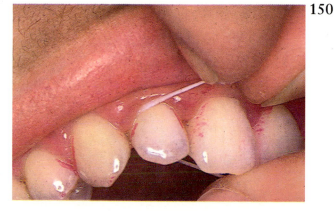

149   Dental floss—finger position. The ends of the floss are wound around the middle finger of each hand, leaving the thumb and forefinger free to guide the working section. The floss is passed through the contact point with a bucco-lingual sliding action. An alternative method is to take a length of about 30 cm and knot it to form a loop. This can then be wrapped round the fingers of each hand and guided between the teeth.

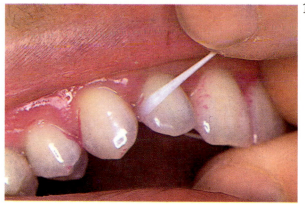

150   Dental floss—distal aspects. The distal surface is cleaned by bringing the floss to the base of the gingival sulcus. The need to take the floss to the base of the sulcus with each wiping movement is stressed.

151   Dental floss—vertical action The floss is tensioned against the distal surface and moved up and down using a vertical wiping action. This is repeated until the surface is free of stained plaque.

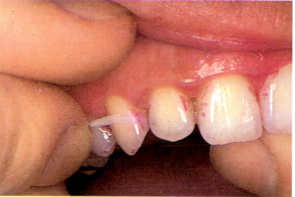

152   Dental floss—mesial aspect. The floss is then brought across the embrasure to clean the mesial tooth surface, this time applying tension in the opposite direction and the same vertical wiping action is used. Each interspace is then cleaned in the same way in a systematic order. Care should be taken not to damage the soft tissues.

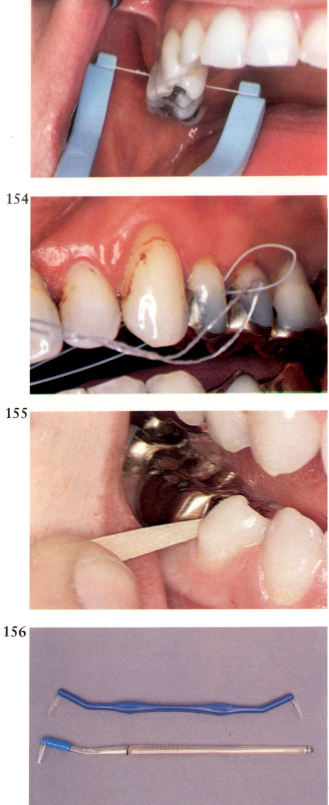

153 **Floss holder** Where difficulty is experienced in reaching the back of the mouth a floss holder may be used.

154 **Floss threaders.** Floss threaders should be used for cleaning between the retainers and pontics of bridgework and for cleaning between splinted teeth. Lengths of specially prepared floss, superfloss, are available with a stiffened end to use as a threader and with an expanded, foam-textured section for cleaning irregular surfaces.[13]

155 **Wood sticks** Triangular-shaped interdental wood sticks are an alternative method of interproximal cleaning. In some respects they are almost as effective as floss, and they are easier to use. A variety of sizes is available and an appropriate one should be selected for the size of the interproximal spaces. The wood sticks are used with a bucco-lingual rubbing action against the interdental tooth surfaces and papillae. The angulation of the wood stick is important and this must be adjusted so that the gingivae on the lingual aspect are not traumatised. Wood sticks are less effective where there are deeper interproximal pockets—dental floss can penetrate these further. The lingual aspects of the embrasures are less well cleaned and a single-tufted brush may be used in addition to reach these areas.[9,14]

156 **Interdental brushes.** Where embrasures are large and the roots have concave surfaces, interdental brushes may be more effective than floss or wood sticks. There are designs with metal or plastic handles, and various sizes of heads are available on some models.[9]

157 Pulsed water jet instruments. These are available from several manufacturers. It has been found that the regular use of water lavage brings about a reduction in gingival inflammation by diluting the concentration of plaque metabolites; modified bacterial cells, however, still remain adhering to the tooth surface.[15] Water jet instruments may be used for cleaning fixed orthodontic appliances and temporary splints, and they are of value to handicapped patients with poor manual dexterity.

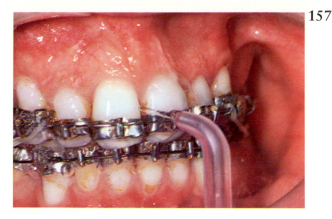

REMOVAL OF PLAQUE-RETAINING FACTORS (see Chapter 10)

Following oral hygiene instruction, all periodontally involved teeth are scaled, root planed and polished, and the margins of restorations which are in contact with the gingiva are smoothed.

CHEMICAL PLAQUE CONTROL

Many different chemical agents have been used in the prevention and treatment of periodontal diseases, with varying degrees of success. Drugs which have been used systemically have included antibiotics. Drugs which have been used topically include antiseptics, enzymes, oxidising agents and surfactants. These topical applications have involved the use of mouthwashes, tooth pastes and gels, sub-gingival irrigation and various techniques which allow the application of drugs sub-gingivally, where they are slowly released.

Dentifrices with anti-plaque activity are being developed. For example a dentifrice containing zinc citrate and a non-anionic antimicrobial agent Triclosan proved effective at maintaining gingival health over a 12 month period compared with a control dentifrice.[16]

158 Chlorhexidine mouthwash. Mouthwashes of various sorts have been used for years but relatively few have proved to be effective for controlling plaque in the treatment of chronic periodontal disease or caries. Although various antiseptics have been shown to be active against a wide spectrum of oral bacteria, one of the essential properties often lacking seems to be substantivity, i.e., absorption into the surfaces of the oral mucosa and teeth.

It has been shown[17] that a 0.2 per cent solution of chlorhexidine used as a mouthwash was effective in preventing plaque growth on clean tooth surfaces in the absence of pocketing. As the antiseptic is absorbed on to mucosa, pellicle and tooth surfaces, it is effective for 8 to 12 hours after rinsing. Despite this promising finding, few studies have shown that mouthwashes incorporating antiseptics are effective in treating established disease; this may be because mouthwashes do not penetrate very far into periodontal pockets.[18]

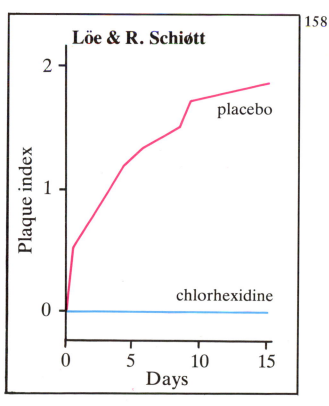

Chlorhexidine mouthwash has beneficial effects in controlling plaque after oral and periodontal surgery and in mouths with painful gingiva or mucosa, for example in aphthous ulceration. In addition, it has been found useful for patients who are mentally or physically handicapped.

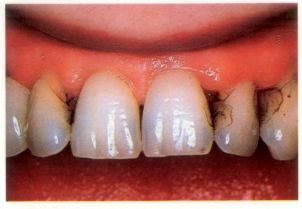

159 Chlorhexidine stain. The main problem with the use of chlorhexidine is that a brown stain tends to form on the teeth. The solution has a bitter taste, and some patients complain of a 'burning' sensation from the mucosa after a period of using the mouthwash.

Other antiseptics, for example Listerine, Sanguinarine or the Keye's method (bicarbonate of soda with hydrogen peroxide) have been the subject of recent research. Compared to chlorhexidine these antiseptics have been found to be less effective at controlling plaque and inflammation. Side effects have also been reported.[19,20]

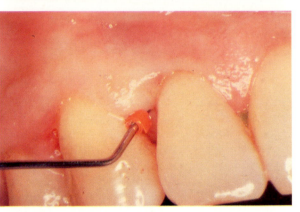

160 Sub-gingival drug application. Because mouthwashes do not penetrate pockets, a variety of delivery systems have been tried to investigate the effect of drugs sub-gingivally. Such systems have included the use of sub-gingival irrigation and the application of drugs using a slow release system. Short-term benefits have been described but there are no studies to show long-term benefits. Future developments may include techniques based on these principles for the treatment of localised residual pockets.

REINFORCEMENT OF PLAQUE CONTROL

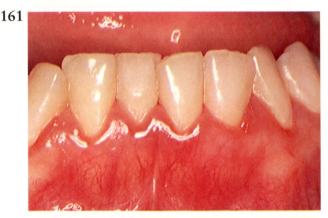

161 Gingivitis—partial resolution after 4 weeks of treatment. Progress is reassessed at each visit. It is now 4 weeks after the start of this patient's treatment (see **140** and **141**). She is shown the improvement in the periodontal condition and given encouragement.

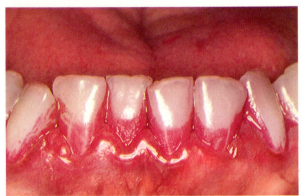

162 Plaque control—reassessed by disclosing agent. Plaque deposits are disclosed and the sites requiring particular attention emphasised. Oral hygiene procedures are again demonstrated, the patient's own performance observed and any necessary correction given.

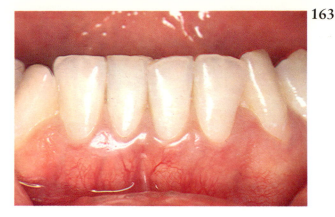

163   Resolution of gingivitis now complete. Over a 4-month period there has been resolution of inflammation as a result of the excellent plaque control maintained by the patient. She must be informed about the need to maintain this high standard of oral hygiene. At recall visits co-operation must be assessed and the instruction reinforced.

DENTAL HYPERSENSITIVITY—CAUSES AND TREATMENT

During the early stages of periodontal treatment gingival recession is a common occurrence, as a result of the reduction in both oedema and vasodilation of the soft tissues. If consequently dentine is exposed to the oral environment, hypersensitivity to hot and cold substances or to cold air is likely to occur. At the cervical margin the developmental relationship of enamel and cementum, and hence the degree of coverage of the underlying dentine is variable;[21] in addition incorrect brushing techniques or caries may be other factors causing dentine to be exposed. Treatment of dental hypersensitivity consists of ensuring that toothbrushing procedures are efficient, but yet not traumatic to the tissues. The application of fluoride varnish is usually beneficial. The patient may be advised to use desensitising toothpaste. Dentifrices containing silica particles have been found to occlude the dentinal tubules mechanically.[22,23,24]

Scaling

If plaque control procedures are not ideal, calcified deposits tend to form on the teeth. Calculus may form both supragingivally and subgingivally. Supragingival calculus is pale yellow or light brown in colour and is found most commonly on surfaces of teeth in proximity to the duct orifices of the parotid and submandibular salivary glands; for example, on the buccal aspects of the maxillary first molar and on the lingual aspects of the mandibular incisor teeth. Supragingival calculus is formed by the deposition of calcium and phosphate ions from saliva.

Subgingival calculus is dark grey or black and is formed from crevicular fluid. It is relatively thin and tends to be attached tenaciously to the tooth surface. This characteristic, together with the hardness of the deposit, usually necessitates heavy force having to be applied when scaling subgingival calculus.

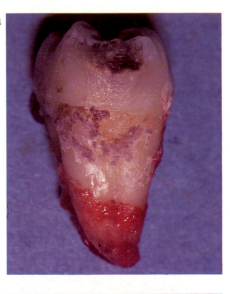

164a

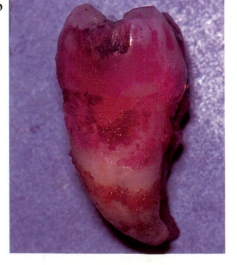

164b

THE DISTRIBUTION OF DEPOSITS AND THE ROLE OF LOCAL ANALGESIA IN SCALING AND ROOT PLANING

164a　Extracted tooth with calculus. This tooth has been extracted because of severe periodontitis, and extensive calculus deposits are present on the affected root surface. Before extraction, the greater part of these deposits had been covered by the gingiva which had extended to within about 1 mm of the enamel-cement junction. The extent and relative inaccessibility of subgingival calculus makes complete removal difficult, especially in deeper pockets.[1]

164b　Disclosed plaque on calculus. The calculus deposits are covered with a layer of plaque and this has been stained with disclosing solution. There is a narrow clear zone on the root, apical to the stained deposits, which represents the previous attachment site of the junctional epithelium. On this tooth it can be seen that the deposits extend apically to the level of the junctional epithelium at the base of the pocket. Insertion of a scaling instrument to this level is liable to be painful, especially where the pockets are deep and access is restricted, therefore local analgesia is recommended for treating deep periodontal pockets. When working under local analgesia, however, care must be taken not to cause excessive trauma, especially at sites with minimal periodontal involvement, as several studies have noted loss of attachment following scaling or root planing of shallow pockets.[2,3]

ASSESSMENT AND THE DETECTION OF CALCULUS

165   Periodontitis with 5 to 6 mm pockets.
Pockets of 5 to 6 mm are present in the mandibular anterior region of this 48-year-old man. He had been aware of bleeding from his gums on brushing and had been told that he had halitosis.

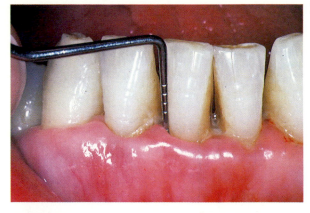

165

166   Detection of subgingival calculus—coronal edge. Subgingival calculus is detected using a fine probe. The coronal edge of the labial deposit is evident as a hard ledge which interferes with the apical movement of the probe.

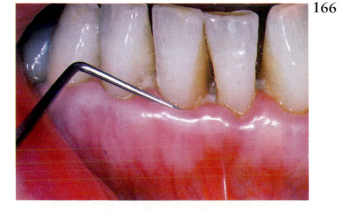

166

167   Detection of subgingival calculus—apical edge. The probe tip is then disengaged from the coronal edge of the calculus and is moved apically over the surface of the deposit, enabling the slight roughness of texture to be felt. The probe is now registering the apical edge of the calculus which is detected by the deviation of the probe tip as it passes from the jutting out calculus on to the root surface.

167

168   Detection of subgingival calculus interproximally. The interproximal surface is being probed in the same way for the presence of subgingival calculus. The probe is held with a light grasp so that the relatively slight deflection at the edges of the deposit can be felt.
    The presence of deposits can also be confirmed as the instrument is moved coronally in the opposite direction by again passing it over the root, thus enabling the presence of an apical positive edge and a coronal negative edge to be recognised.

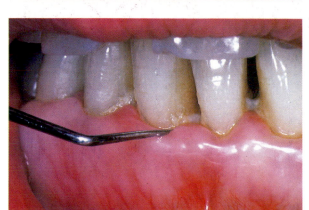

168

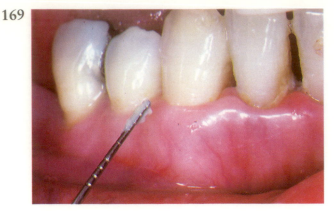

169   **Demonstration of plaque retained on calculus.** The presence of plaque on these calculus deposits is being demonstrated by the removal of a sample on a probe. The significance of calculus in the aetiology of periodontal disease is that it causes the retention of plaque deposits on its irregular surface, preventing adequate plaque control. The edges of the deposit also hinder the effective use of dental floss.

REMOVAL OF DEPOSITS—ULTRASONIC AND MECHANICAL SCALERS

Research work has indicated that the effectiveness of removal of deposits and the resolution of inflammation is similar after instrumentation either by hand or ultrasonic instruments. Finishing procedures, however, may best be performed by hand instruments as these allow greater tactile definition of the surface being treated.[4,5,2,6]

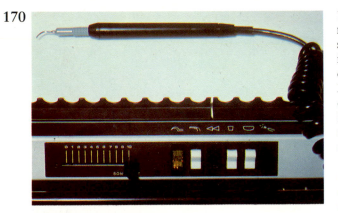

170   **Ultrasonic scaler.** Removal of deposits is made easier and quicker by using an ultrasonic scaler and many dental units now include this instrument as a built-in feature.[7] The control box delivers an alternating current of approximately 25,000 cycles per second to the handpiece, which contains a water-cooled coil.[8] Within this coil there is either a stack of metal plates activated by magnetostrictive effect to produce vibrations, or a quartz-like crystal activated by piezo-electric effect.

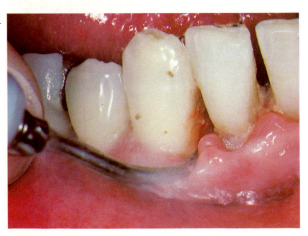

171   **Ultrasonic scaler in use.** An antiseptic mouthwash should be used before instrumentation in order to reduce the bacteria in the aerosol spray.[9,10] An ultrasonic scaling tip is removing subgingival calculus and plaque from the mesial surface of the canine tooth. Removal of deposits may be achieved by several mechanisms. (1) mechanical vibration of the tip; (2) release of ultrasonic energy at the change of phase at the boundary between calculus and cementum; (3) the cavitation effect may be a source of energy: vapour bubbles formed in the water spray by the rapid movements of the tip implode with the release of energy.[8,11]

Mechanical scalers which are powered by the compressed air supply are also available but vibrate at below ultrasonic frequency. Preliminary reports indicate that they compare favourably with ultrasonic scalers.[12]

MANUAL SCALERS

172   Chisel scaler—supragingival scaling. This hand instrument is termed a chisel or push scaler, and several widths of tip are available. It is used to remove interproximal supragingival deposits by means of a horizontal cleaving action and is particularly valuable for treating narrow embrasures, where access of more bulky instruments is impossible. It is easier to use in the anterior region but may also be used posteriorly. The instrument may be used to reduce overhanging margins by repeated paring actions (see **358** and **359**); frequent sharpening is essential during this procedure.

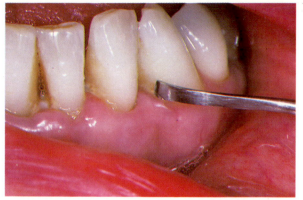

172

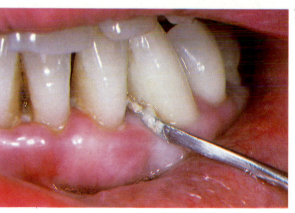

173

173   Chisel scaler—gauging pocket depth. The chisel scaler can also be used for subgingival scaling interproximally. The instrument is first inserted interproximally and moved down the root surface until the level of the soft tissue attachment is felt and, having gauged this, the scaler is withdrawn to the line angle maintaining this depth.

174   Chisel scaler—subgingival scaling. The scaler is now re-introduced at the level previously gauged, with force being exerted against the tooth to cleave the calculus from its surface. The instrument is not suitable for the deeper aspects of complex pockets.

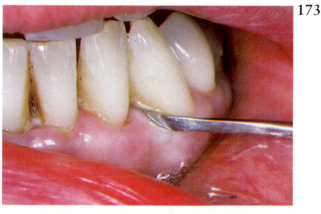

174

SICKLE SCALERS

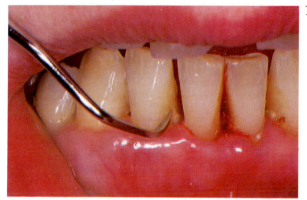

175

175   Sickle scaler in use. This is used mainly for removal of deposits where pockets are relatively shallow. The pointed tip is useful for cleaning the embrasures near the contact points. Suitable instruments have been designed which permit access to all parts of the mouth. The tip of the scaler is introduced gently into the pocket until the apical edge of the calculus is felt. Force is applied to the blade horizontally against the tooth surface, and the instrument is then withdrawn vertically, cleaving calculus from the tooth.

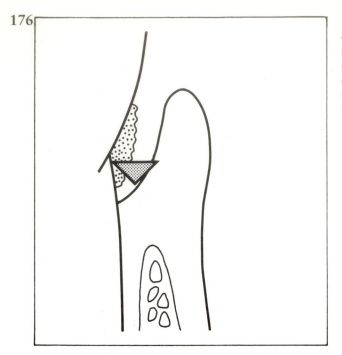

176 Sickle scaler—diagram. The triangular cross-section of this instrument may make it less suitable for use subgingivally where pockets are deeper, the depth of the blade tending to prevent the cutting edge reaching the apical extent of the deposits. The non-working edges may also traumatise the lining of the pocket.

PERIODONTAL HOES

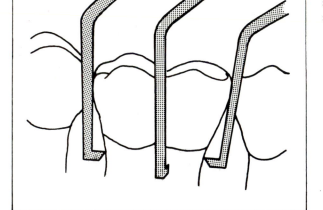

177 Set of periodontal hoes. A set of hoes comprises four instruments, giving access to all surfaces of the teeth. (Hoe on lingual aspect not shown.)

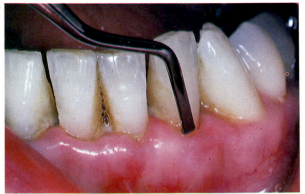

178 Periodontal hoe—blade about to the inserted into pocket. The tip of the hoe is passed over the deposit on the root surface until the base of the pocket is felt. The tip of the instrument is bulky and may not be applicable when the tissues of the pocket are closely applied to the tooth, in which case a finer instrument is indicated—for example, a curette.

179 Periodontal hoe at base of pocket. The shank of the instrument should be in contact with the crown to achieve the correct angulation of the blade to the tooth. Before the scaling stroke, firm pressure is applied to the blade against the root.

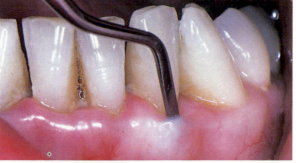

179

180 Calculus being removed by the periodontal hoe. Maintaining this pressure against the root, the instrument is withdrawn, thus cleaving calculus from a narrow, vertical strip of the surface. The short cutting edge of the hoe results in considerable pressure being applied to a restricted area, hence it is very useful for the removal of tenacious, hard deposits. Consecutive strokes should be overlapped circumferentially to achieve complete instrumentation.

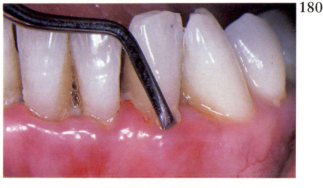

180

181 Periodontal hoe applied interproximally. In the interproximal region the shank will have to be angled to permit the blade to be applied to the root surface below the contact point. Where embrasures are wider this angulation may be nearly horizontal.

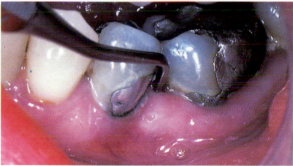

181

182 Limitations on the use of periodontal hoes. The position of the cutting edge relative to the end of the instrument may prevent the root surface at the bottom of the pocket being treated; in addition, the narrow cutting edge tends to leave vertical grooves in the root surface. It is necessary to use a finishing instrument, for example a curette, subsequently.

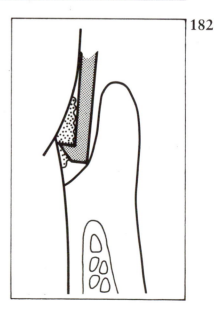

182

CURETTES

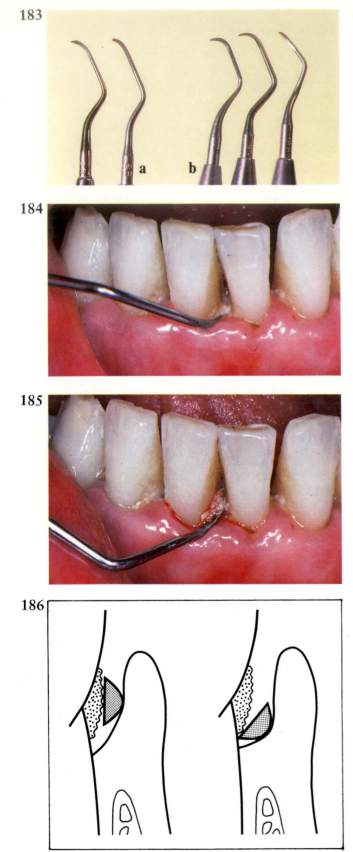

183

184

185

186

183 A selection of periodontal curettes (a) Universal; (b) Gracey. Usually, paired sets of anterior and posterior instruments will suffice, but additional instruments may be required for particular problems. There are various sizes of blade; heavy ones are used for dense deposits and finer ones for finishing. Most curettes have an inner and an outer cutting edge which is continuous around the tip—these are Universal curettes.

Gracey curettes have only one edge, the non-working aspect being blunted so that the soft tissues are not traumatised. As a result, however, a greater number of instruments is needed to gain access to all the tooth surfaces.

184 Insertion of curette into pocket. The tip of the instrument is insinuated into the pocket and the blade passed down the root until the base of the pocket is felt. Firm pressure is applied to the blade against the root surface as a preliminary to the cutting stroke.

185 Withdrawal of curette. The firm pressure is maintained as the blade is withdrawn, thus cleaving the deposits from the root. This instrument has a long cutting edge and so achieves a broader zone of treated root surface per stroke than the hoe, hence the curette acts as a useful finishing instrument.

186 Angle of application of curette. This diagram illustrates the angle of application, rake angle, of the blade to the root surface. When the rake angle is small there is a burnishing effect on the root with minimal damage to soft tissue. As the rake angle is increased, a cutting action is produced with greater removal of hard tissue but the change in angulation results in greater soft tissue trauma from the opposite edge. The diagram also shows that access for the blade usually can be achieved to the full depth of the pocket.

187 Horizontal action with curette. The curette may also be applied to the tooth surface with a horizontal action, but care must be taken to avoid damage to the epithelium at the base of the pocket. This technique is used commonly on the marginal aspects and where there are restorations which might be damaged by vertical strokes.

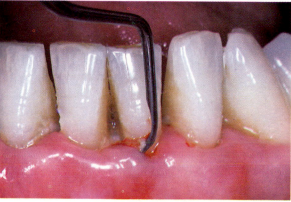

188 Deposits being removed. The tip of the instrument is guided along the base of the pocket so that complete removal of deposits is achieved.

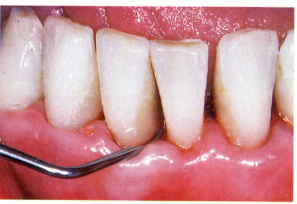

Root planing

189 Curette being used for root planing. Following the removal of calculus from all affected surfaces and having confirmed this by probing, it may be considered necessary to root plane contaminated root surfaces. Research into contaminants within the superficial layer of cementum on periodontally involved teeth has indicated that substances are present which may retard the growth and adhesion of host cells.[13,14,15,16,17] Following the removal of deposits, the underlying cementum should be planed meticulously to remove irritants from the surface layer. The planing of the contaminated roots should be continued until the surfaces feel completely smooth.[18] Research is continuing to find less traumatic ways to remove the irritants.[19,20,21] The surfaces should be washed thoroughly after root planing to remove debris and contaminants. The aim is to encourage the formation of a new junctional epithelium (see Appendix 6).

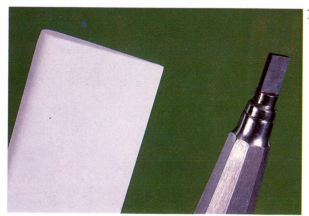

190 Sharpening stone and tungsten carbide sharpener. Scaling causes considerable deformation and blunting of the cutting edges of instruments, reducing their effectiveness for root planing.[22,23,24,25] It may be useful to have a sterilised sharpening stone on the instrument tray, so that curettes can be sharpened immediately before the actual root planing phase of treatment.

Polishing

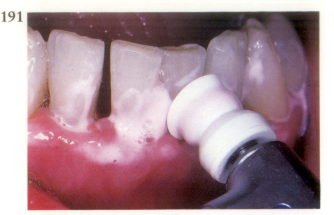

191 **Polishing tooth surfaces.** The crown and root surfaces are being polished with a paste containing fluoride. The choice of abrasive for achieving a smooth tooth surface does not seem to be critical.[26] A rubber cup will polish the surfaces up to about 1 mm subgingivally on the marginal aspects but access cannot be gained to interproximal surfaces using cups or brushes.

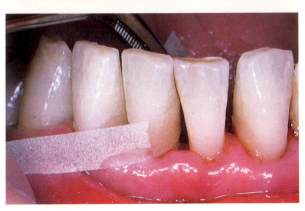

192 **Abrasive polishing strip.** A polishing strip is used interproximally with horizontal action, the width of the strip being dependent on the space available.

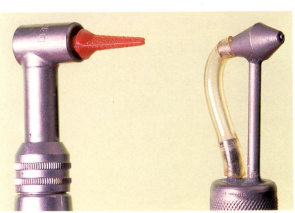

193 **Reciprocating handpiece and air/powder instrument for polishing.** A reciprocating handpiece with triangular insert and polishing paste may be used as an alternative to the abrasive strip.

The recently introduced air polishing instruments utilise an air-propelled jet of sodium bicarbonate powder surrounded by a concentric jet of water. Although these instruments may be of value supragingivally for the removal of stain and deposits from enamel, several studies have reported rapid erosion of cementum and dentine and of the resin component of composite restorations.[27,28] There is also the disadvantage of contamination of both operator and environment with sodium bicarbonate and micro-organisms during their use.

RESPONSES OF THE TISSUES TO TREATMENT

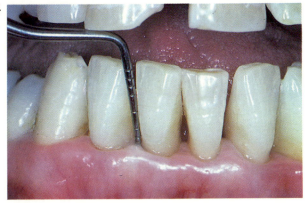

194 **Probing 4 months after start of treatment.** The patient has been attending at intervals of about 2 months to reinforce oral hygiene procedures. Four months after the initial treatment, there has been resolution of inflammation; pocket depths on probing are 2 mm or less. The reduction in pocketing is attributable to the shrinkage of the tissue, resulting from a reduction in oedema and vascularity and to greater resistance of the junctional epithelium to probe penetration. Another improvement noted was a reduction in the mobility of the teeth. Changes in mobility with healing have been attributed to a reduction in width of the periodontal ligament and an increase in bone density.[29]

11 GINGIVECTOMY

The general indications for periodontal surgery are given in Appendix 8 and these considerations are applied in deciding on the appropriateness of any periodontal treatment plan involving surgical procedures. The gingivectomy procedure is used to introduce the concepts of periodontal surgery, as the objectives are relatively simple and can act as a basis to establish the principles of the surgical treatment of pockets. It is not, however, the most frequently applied periodontal surgical procedure.

INDICATIONS FOR GINGIVECTOMY

195   Gingivitis. Gingivectomy is sometimes the surgical procedure of choice where there is severe gingival hyperplasia. Enlargement of the gingival tissue, especially in the presence of severe irregularity and distortion of the surface contour, would create practical difficulties if a flap procedure were contemplated. The procedure enables pockets to be eliminated and, simultaneously, gingival tissues to be contoured, by means of a tapered incision excising the hyperplastic tissue at the level of the base of the pocket.

196   Periodontitis. Periodontitis results in loss of attachment and destruction of supporting tissues. Provided there is an adequate zone of attached gingiva apical to the proposed line of incision, however, a gingivectomy may be considered as an alternative to a flap procedure (see Chapter 12). Gingivectomy has a limited application as it is contra-indicated where there are pockets extending beyond the muco-gingival junction, or where there are infra-bony defects (see **214** and **215**).[1]

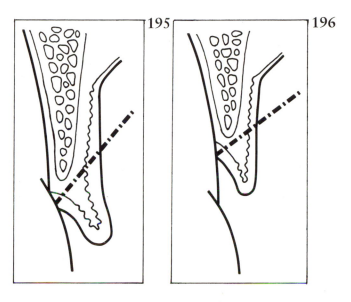

OPERATIVE TECHNIQUE

197   Infiltration of local analgesic. Topical analgesic was applied before the injections. Local infiltration of 2 per cent lignocaine with adrenaline 1 in 80,000 is being administered. For the labial infiltration, the initial injection is made into the submucosa of the vestibule and the needle is then passed horizontally through the tissues at the level of the apices of the teeth. Using this technique, multiple infiltration injections are avoided. On the palatal aspect, local infiltrations are made according to which area is being treated. In the mandible, nerve-block analgesia may be used but, subsequently, there is greater blood loss unless supplementary local infiltration techniques are used.[2]

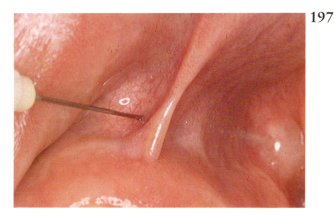

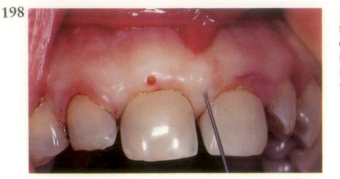

198 Additional infiltrations. When the first infiltrations have taken effect, additional injections of local analgesic are made into the papillae and marginal gingiva. The consequent vasoconstriction results in less bleeding and hence, improved visibility during surgery.

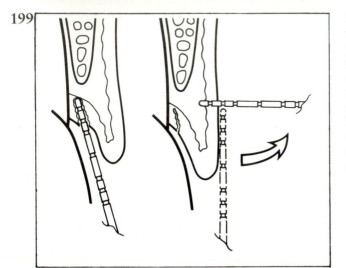

199 to 201 Measuring and marking the levels of the pockets. Pockets are measured with a periodontal probe and this measurement is transferred to the outer aspect of the gingiva, where the probe is up-ended and a puncture point made with the tip of the instrument. By repeating these measurements across the operative site, a series of bleeding points marking the base of the pockets is achieved. An alternative method is to use pocket marking forceps; however, these are difficult to apply interproximally.

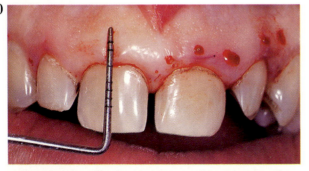

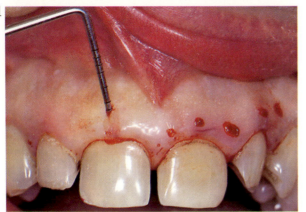

202 Gingivectomy incision (Blake knife). The gingivectomy incision is commenced at a papilla, and is made at a level of about 2 to 4 mm apically to the bleeding points which mark the base of the pockets. The position of the incision is determined by the thickness of the tissue and the blade is angled so that a tapered margin will be achieved.[3] The incision is being made with a Blake gingivectomy knife. This instrument has an angled shank and is one of several similar types designed to hold a disposable scalpel blade. The factory-sharpened edge reduces drag to a minimum and the blade can be renewed during the operation as necessary.

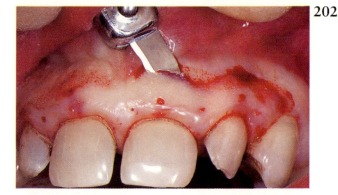

202

203 Gingivectomy incision (Kirkland knife). The incision on this side is being made with a Kirkland knife. There are several types of similar instruments, each having an integral blade which requires to be sharpened before, and sometimes during, the surgical procedure.

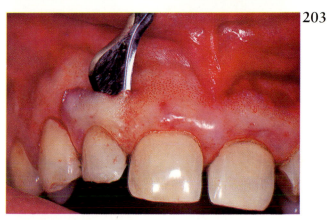

203

204 Interproximal incision (Blake knife). After the main incisions have been made, the interproximal incisions are completed with a Blake knife and a number 11 blade. At each site the incision is taken disto-mesially across the papilla and as far interproximally as the embrasure space will permit.

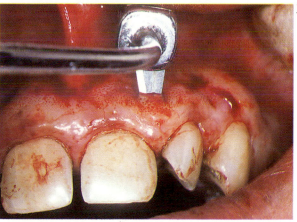

204

205 Interproximal incision (Goldman Fox knife). A variety of instruments is available for the interproximal incisions; here a Goldman Fox knife is used. Similar incisions are carried out on the palatal aspect.

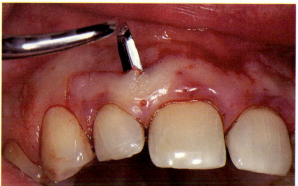

205

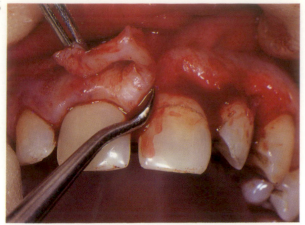

206 Removal of redundant tissue. When the incisions have been completed, the redundant gingival tissue can be removed with a relatively heavy-bladed instrument, for example, a Cumine scaler or Prichard curette. If the incisions have been made accurately, the removal of this tissue should be easy and relatively few tags should remain.

207

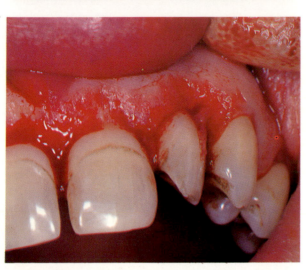

207 Debridement. Epithelial tags and chronically inflamed connective tissues have been removed by curettage. The root surfaces are now to be treated by scaling and root planing to remove residual deposits and contaminated cementum. Copious irrigation with saline is indicated to wash away this debris and enhance visibility.

208

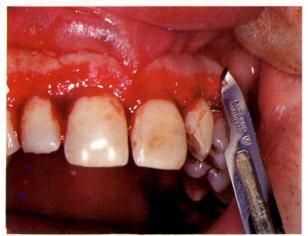

208 Modifying the contour. The contour of the incision should be refined and blended with the adjoining intact tissue. The bevel of the incision can be enhanced if necessary at this stage. The contouring procedure, or gingivoplasty, is being performed with a scalpel using a scraping action. Other techniques include the use of gingivoplasty clippers or rotating diamond stones.

209 and 210   Checking pocket elimination. Both the labial and palatal aspects are now probed to ensure that the pockets have been eliminated. If necessary, further tissue can be excised locally to modify any incompletely treated pockets and to blend the contour with the adjoining tissue.

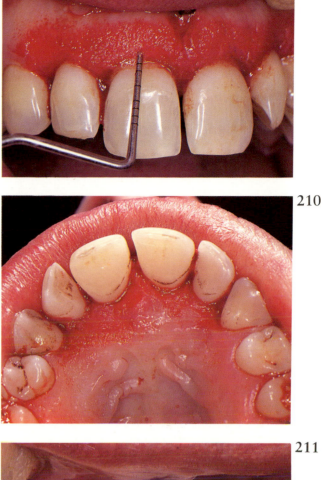

211   Periodontal dressing. A periodontal dressing is necessary after gingivectomy to protect the wound surface from trauma during healing and to reduce pain. Several dressings are available; they should not contain potentially harmful or irritating agents such as asbestos fibres or eugenol. The margin of the dressing must not be overextended. Pressure should be applied to the interproximal regions of the dressing with a cotton wool pledget or cotton bud covered with petroleum jelly, thus achieving adaptation to the interdental spaces. A figure-of-eight floss ligature ensures increased retention for the dressing. The patient is advised to use an antiseptic mouthwash, for example, 0.1 per cent chlorhexidine twice daily.

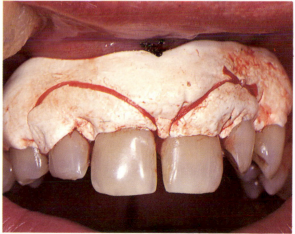

212

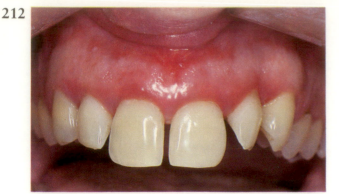

212 **Postoperative healing 3 weeks after surgery.** One week after surgery the dressings are removed. The clinician should ensure that all traces of dressing and all deposits, especially in proximity to the healing tissues, have been cleared. The antiseptic mouthwash is continued for 2 to 4 weeks after periodontal surgery.

The healing is assessed 3 weeks after surgery. The epithelialisation of the wound has progressed very well, but further keratinisation of the epithelium and maturation of the connective tissue has yet to occur.

213

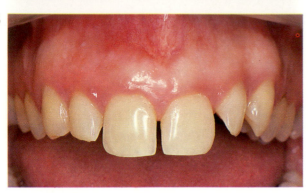

213 **Healing completed.** Three months after surgery there is satisfactory tissue contour, the pockets have been eliminated and there is no evidence of inflammation. The patient is maintaining excellent oral hygiene but it is mandatory that long-term follow-up is maintained at regular intervals.

12 INVERSE BEVEL PERIODONTAL FLAP PROCEDURES

The general indications for periodontal surgery are considered in Appendix 8. Probably the most commonly used procedure is the inverse bevel periodontal flap because of its versatility. The incision may be designed so that virtually all of the gingiva is conserved or, in contrast, it may be designed to thin or reduce the coronal height of the tissue. After flap reflection, excellent access is provided for the removal of deposits from the root surfaces, for root planing and for the treatment of osseous defects. The position of the flap when suturing can be modified to achieve a varying degree of root coverage or exposure postoperatively. The detailed techniques for the inverse bevel flap procedure are described in *A Colour Atlas of Periodontal Surgery*.[1]

214 Pockets extending apically to the muco-gingival junction. A conservative inverse bevel incision at the crest of the gingiva enables the maximum width of keratinised gingiva to be retained (see **361**). If the pocket is shallow an intra-sulcular incision can be used.

215 Use of the incision to improve access. The use of the inverse bevel incision offers excellent access to the involved root surfaces and for the treatment of any osseous defects (see **252** to **254**).

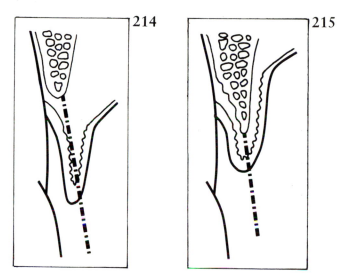

214

215

OPERATIVE TECHNIQUE

216 Residual pockets after the plaque control phase. After completion of the plaque control phase of treatment, this patient has residual interproximal pockets of about 5 mm. There is bleeding on probing, indicating residual inflammation. An inverse bevel flap procedure is to be used to eliminate these pockets but, at the same time, it is required to conserve most of the existing labial and buccal keratinised gingiva as the pockets approach the level of the muco-gingival junction.[2]

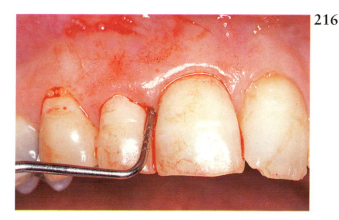

216

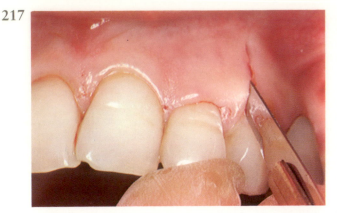

217 **The relieving incision.** The region being treated has been infiltrated with analgesic. A vertical relieving incision is used at the extremity of the operative site. This incision is not always required but may be used to improve access or to facilitate apical repositioning of the flap. The relieving incision is commenced at the line angle of the tooth, where the papilla joins the marginal gingiva; adequate access is thus obtained for treatment of the associated interproximal region. It is important not to make the incision on the marginal gingivae as this is liable to result in a notched outline after healing.

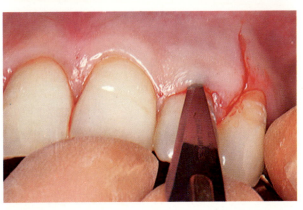

218 **The inverse bevel incision.** The inverse bevel incision is made with a scalloped outline holding the blade at an angle of 10° to the long axes of the teeth so that, subsequently, there will be adequate coverage of interproximal bone. The incision should be made through the full thickness of the soft tissue to the underlying bone. The positioning of the incision relative to the gingival margin may be varied: (1) an intra-sulcular incision or an incision at the gingival crest may be used where the pocketing at a particular site is relatively shallow and the tissue quality is good (see **361**); (2) an incision to thin hyperplastic tissue may be made just apical to the crest of the gingiva, as in this patient; (3) to eliminate deeper pockets in the presence of fibrous hyperplasia, the incision is made a predetermined distance from the gingival margin (see **236**).

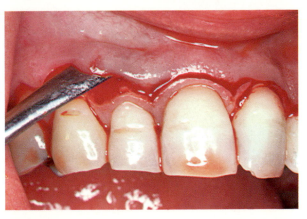

219 **Elevation of the flap.** The flap is now elevated, the mucoperiosteum usually being separated from the bone by blunt dissection. An alternative technique is the use of sharp dissection, either with the purpose of thinning the flap or to leave a layer of periosteum covering the bone. This 'split-flap' procedure is only applicable where the mucoperiosteum is sufficiently thick to permit its dissection. Retention of periosteum by this technique may be indicated where there is a dehiscence or fenestration of the alveolar bone, or where the marginal bone is thin, making it imperative to minimise postsurgical bone resorption.[3]

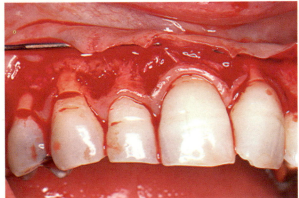

220 **Before curettage.** Having elevated the flap, the residual hyperplastic tissue and the lining of the pocket wall remain attached to the bone and root surfaces. Prolonged inflammation has resulted in the proliferation of epithelium, connective tissue and blood vessels which have to be removed by curettage.

221 Curettage. The redundant tissue is being removed. The main bulk of the tissue is separated from the bone and root surface with a relatively broad-bladed instrument. A supplementary intra-crevicular incision may be used if the tissue is very tenacious. Remaining tags and inflammatory granulation tissue are removed with fine curettes.

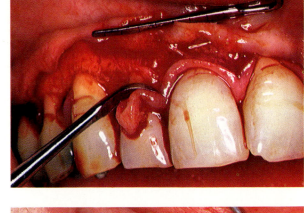

221

222 Root planing. The root surfaces are being planed to remove the residual calculus and contaminated cementum. It has been found that the surface of cementum on periodontally involved roots contains toxins and other substances that may interfere with healing (see Appendix 6). All exposed root surfaces are root planed with sharpened curettes until they feel smooth and hard.

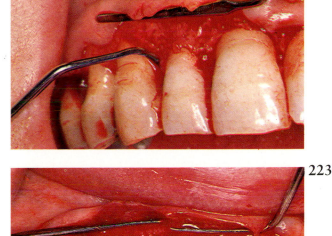

222

223 Assessment of bone contours The bone contour is assessed; in this patient no osseous defects are present. Before suturing, debris is removed by washing with isotonic saline using a disposable syringe.

223

224 Palatal aspect. Curettage has also been completed on this aspect. Palatally the inverse bevel incision has been made with an enhanced scallop to eliminate pockets on the mid-palatal margins. Emphasis had been placed on producing a thinned flap by sharp dissection so that the resulting tapered, scalloped outline would just cover the bone margins, but with minimal overlap on to the root surface.

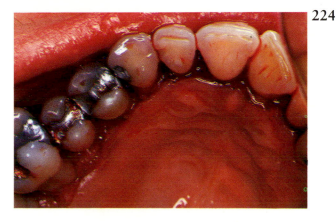

224

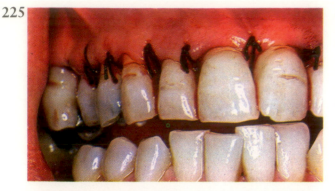

225 Interrupted sutures. The positioning of the flap at the time of suturing is determined by the need to achieve maximum coverage of the roots for aesthetic reasons or, in regions that are less easy for the patient to clean, the objective may be to expose the involved root surfaces to a greater degree to aid plaque control (see **230**).

For this patient, who does not normally show the cervical region of the maxillary anterior teeth, the flap has been repositioned apically by about 1 mm. The tension in the interrupted sutures was adjusted to allow for the required degree of apical repositioning. Various types of suturing are shown in Appendix 11.

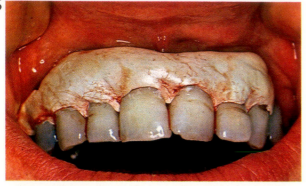

226 The periodontal dressing. The labial flap was held under slight pressure at the desired position for about 5 minutes, so that a fibrin clot would develop and tack the soft tissue to the bone. A firm periodontal dressing was used to stabilise the apically repositioned flap. Dressings are not required for a replaced flap procedure when the flap is not elevated beyond the muco-gingival junction. An antiseptic mouthwash should again be used during the preliminary healing phase to keep the area clean.

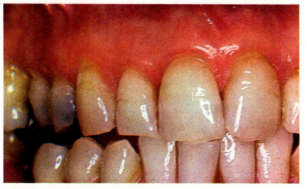

227 Reassessment at 6 weeks—labial aspect. The sutures were removed 1 week after surgery, the teeth being carefully cleaned to remove deposits. The patient was then reassessed 2 weeks later. The accumulation of irritants must be prevented, especially during the preliminary healing phase. Six weeks after surgery a physiological tissue contour has been achieved, the patient having maintained a good standard of oral hygiene. Any areas where plaque deposits are not being removed should be shown to the patient and instruction given. The increased area of root surface exposed by surgery often causes initial problems; cleaning and reinforcement of plaque control is essential.

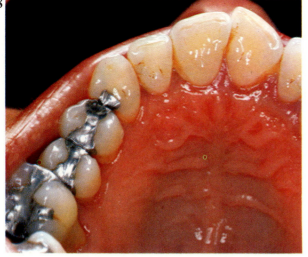

228 Reassessment at 6 weeks—palatal aspect. On the palatal aspect a satisfactory soft tissue contour has been achieved. There is a generalised sulcus depth of 2 mm.

On completion of the surgical phase of treatment, the patient enters the maintenance phase. Recall for regular plaque control is essential and the frequency of such visits is gauged by successive recordings of plaque levels and any recurrence of inflammation.

MODIFICATIONS OF THE INVERSE BEVEL FLAP

229 Diagram to illustrate various incisions. The level at which the inverse bevel incision is made depends on the local anatomy and on the degree of periodontal destruction.

Buccal aspect
Where there is a limited width of gingiva, as much of this tissue should be retained as possible. The incision, therefore, is made close to the gingival margin so that most of the keratinised tissue is conserved.

Palatal aspect
The palatal aspect is invested by keratinised gingival tissue with a thick connective tissue corium which extends to the vault. The resilience of this tissue is such that it cannot be readily repositioned apically and, therefore, palatal pockets must be eliminated by excision. The bone level is estimated by probing through the soft tissue at the base of the pocket. A mark is made on the outer aspect of the gingiva 2 mm coronal to the crest of the bone and the

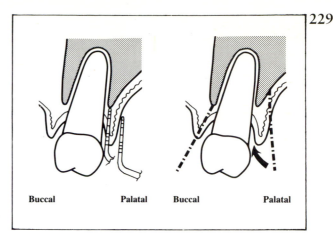

229

Buccal   Palatal   Buccal   Palatal

palatal incision is commenced at this level. If the tissue is thick it may be found easier to make the incision in two stages, an initial outline, followed by a thinning incision. An additional incision (*arrow*) is then made within the sulcus to release the hyperplastic palatal tissue.

230 Positioning of the flap. The positioning of the flap during suturing has been mentioned (see **225**). This is determined by the following factors:
(a) If there is minimal bone loss the flap is replaced at the original level where it will reattach to alveolar bone. Under these circumstances, the inverse bevel procedure offers an alternative to the conventional gingivectomy procedure for the elimination of false pockets.
(b) On the labial aspect of the anterior segment, cosmetic considerations may dictate that the flap be replaced on to the cemental surface of the teeth at the original level in spite of loss of bone. The outcome of this procedure is uncertain as attachment of the flap to cementum cannot be predicted. There is rapid downgrowth of epithelium and the formation of a long junctional epithelial attachment, or possibly reformation of a pocket.
(c) On the palatal aspect the positioning of the inverse bevel incision is designed to result in the removal of the soft tissue wall of the pocket. The flap is thus replaced over the bone with minimal

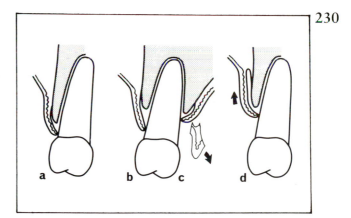

230

a   b   c   d

overlap on to the cemental surfaces of the teeth.
(d) Where there is established bone loss on the buccal aspect, definitive elimination of pockets is obtained by repositioning the flap apically, which enables the existing keratinised gingiva to be conserved.

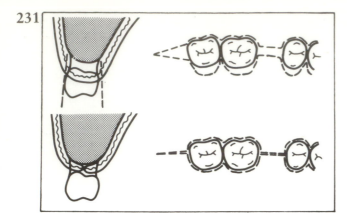

231 Tuberosity, retromolar regions and edentulous ridges. The inverse bevel incision may be extended to treat local pockets associated with the maxillary tuberosity and mandibular retromolar regions, and with edentulous ridges. The former are treated by removing a wedge of tissue distal to the terminal molar. The two lateral incisions for the wedge are made in continuity with the buccal and lingual inverse bevel incisions. The dimensions of the wedge are determined by the thickness of the tissue and the depth of the pocket. Following the removal of this wedge, the flaps may need to be thinned and trimmed to remove excess tissue. Pockets involving an edentulous saddle area are treated by continuing the buccal and lingual inverse bevel incisions along the ridge. The two incisions are made some distance apart, this being determined by the depths of the pockets. When the central block of tissue has been removed the flaps are thinned and trimmed to produce the required contour of ridge.

PRE-RESTORATIVE SURGERY

The use of periodontal surgery before restorative treatment is discussed in Chapter 17. The following surgical sequence is included here as it illustrates various modifications of the inverse bevel procedure.

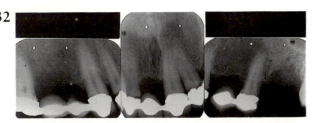

232 Radiographs of bridgework in the maxillary arch. This patient had bridges placed in the maxillary arch about 8 years ago. There is horizontal periodontal bone loss of about 2 to 3 mm. In many places the margins appear less than ideal on the radiographs, there being gaps, overhangs and irregularities.

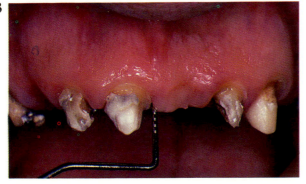

233 Clinical condition after the plaque control phase. The bridgework has been removed to improve access; subsequently, it will be used for temporary cover (see **238**). The response to plaque control has been excellent and there has been considerable improvement in the gingival condition during the preliminary treatment period. There are only relatively few sites where the gingiva bleeds on probing and there is less oedema, but there are 5 mm pockets at most of the abutments including those in proximity to the saddle areas and tuberosity regions. The tissues are thickened with evidence of abundant fibrous tissue.

234   Periodontal condition in the saddle areas.
There is also periodontal bone loss and fibrous
hyperplasia in the region of the saddle areas and
tuberosities. The maxillary arch is to be treated by
periodontal flap surgery so that a healthy
periodontal condition can be achieved, before the
construction of new bridgework.

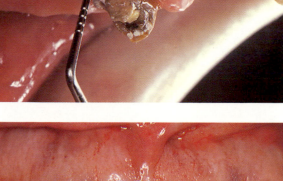

235   After surgery—anterior segment. The labial
segment has been treated by an inverse bevel
incision to thin the excess tissue. The flap has been
apically repositioned to eliminate pockets and
enhance access for achieving good quality margins
for the new bridge. A dressing is to be placed to
retain the flap in the correct position.

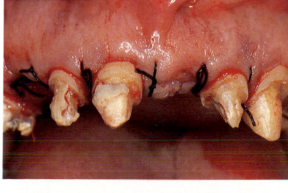

235

236   After surgery—saddle areas and tuberosity.
In the saddle areas and the tuberosity regions the
excess bulk of tissue has been eliminated by the
inverse bevel incisions. On the palatal aspect of the
teeth, the incision was outlined with an enhanced
scallop to remove about 4 mm of tissue height.

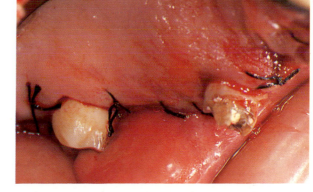

236

237   After surgery—the overall result. The design
of the incisions and the achievement of thinned
flaps on both the facial and palatal aspects has
enabled the hyperplastic tissue to be eliminated. The
margins of the preparations have been exposed, and
the correct relationship of the soft tissues to the
crestal bone has been achieved. Interrupted sutures
have been used to retain the flaps in the correct
position during healing. These will be removed in 1
week.

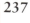

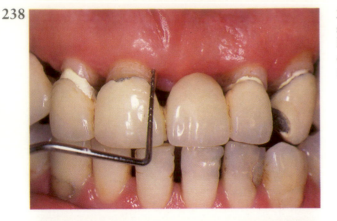

238 Three months after surgery. There has been satisfactory healing over this period. The emphasis has been on regular 3-weekly visits for preventive care. Surgery has provided very good access for the required restorative work.

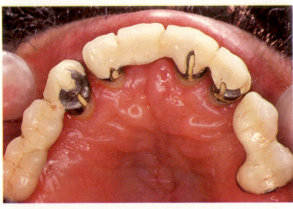

239 Palatal view after surgery. On the palatal aspect the margins of the abutment teeth have been exposed adequately and the tissue contour is now satisfactory.

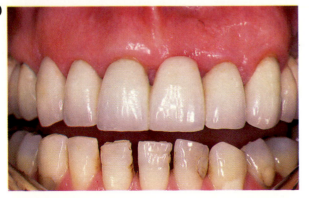

240 The new bridges. Three months after surgery, it was considered that the tissues had matured adequately and the levels of the gingival margins had stabilised; at this stage new bridges were constructed. The margins of the restorations were placed level with the gingiva.

241 Palatal view of new bridges. On the palatal aspect the soft tissues are reacting favourably to the new fixed prostheses. The patient will require continuing preventive maintenance care, with especial emphasis on the particular problems in interproximal cleaning posed by the presence of the pontics. Floss threaders or superfloss are essential and an interdental brush of suitable shape and size may also be helpful (see **154** and **156**).

13 TREATMENT OF OSSEOUS DEFECTS

When periodontal disease has caused a tooth to be affected by bone loss to an equal extent on all surfaces, this is termed horizontal bone loss. Periodontitis, however, may result in uneven bone destruction, vertical bone loss, as a result of a variety of factors. For example, the degree of inflammation induced by local plaque retention will be influenced both by the accessibility of the tooth surface to cleaning procedures and by the presence of any anomaly in tooth form. An additional cause of irregular bone loss is that the alveolus is not homogeneous in structure, being composed of outer dense cortical bone and inner cancellous tissue. The cancellous bone is relatively vascular and may be more susceptible to the destructive agents of periodontitis.

A classification of bone defects is given in Appendix 10. The choice of treatment method is made not only on the basis of the configuration and severity of the bone defect, but also with regard to any local factors such as atypical root morphology or abnormal relationship of adjoining teeth.

The healing of osseous defects may be based on one or more of the following principles:

Repair, in which the aim is to achieve a long junctional epithelial attachment; this may be supplemented by a degree of new bone formation (see Appendix 12(a)).

Surgical elimination of osseous defects, in which the objective is to achieve optimum bone form by the surgical recontouring of osseous defects, thereby reducing the possibility of residual pocketing, for example as a result of the downgrowth of epithelium into infra-bony pockets (see **252** to **255**).

New attachment, which is achieved by the proliferation of new connective tissue from cells in the periodontal ligament to insert into newly formed cementum (see Appendix 12(c)).

Regeneration, which is the reformation of *all* the various components of the periodontium to restore the original anatomy (see Appendix 12(d)).

Extraction of a tooth or root where bone loss is severe may be the treatment of choice (see **282** and **283**; **286** to **293**). Such decisions are best made early in the course of treatment.

REPAIR AFTER ROOT PLANING AND PLAQUE CONTROL

Repair may be achieved by various techniques, the simplest being by root planing with plaque control, and this technique forms the basis for the other more complex procedures. Surgical procedures may be considered subsequently if there is incomplete resolution of inflammation at a site, for example, where there is an osseous defect.

242   Radiograph of bone defect on first molar tooth. This 45-year-old patient has a localised 7 mm pocket on the distal aspect of the mandibular first molar tooth, which was treated by plaque control with root planing. The patient was very co-operative with oral hygiene measures and attended regularly for maintenance treatment, which included subgingival removal of deposits by the clinician especially at the sites with residual pockets.

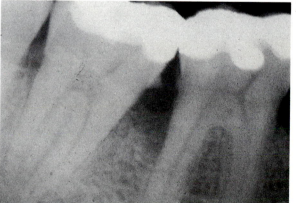

242

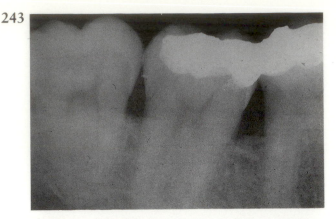

243 Radiograph 4 years later—bone repair.
Assessment 4 years later revealed a reduction of pocket depth to 3 mm. The radiograph indicates that there has been considerable repair of the osseous defect, with consolidation of crestal bone.

The reduction in pocket depth will have been achieved mainly by soft tissue shrinkage and by the formation of a long junctional epithelial attachment. The bone repair seen on the radiograph will have resulted mainly from an increase in bone density. Although after root planing there is an increase in the collagen content of the supracrestal connective tissue with the reduction of inflammation, this is not usually accompanied by a coronal gain in connective tissue attachment.[1]

REPAIR OF AN ACUTE LESION, TREATED SURGICALLY

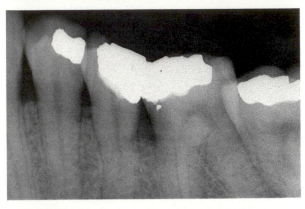

244 Radiograph showing initial bone level. The patient, a 36-year-old female, was being treated by root planing with plaque control. There was originally a 4 mm pocket on the mesial aspect of the mandibular first molar tooth, and the radiograph showed an estimated bone loss of 3 mm.

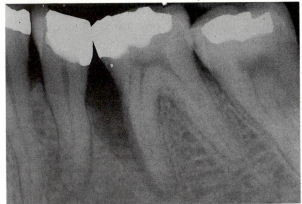

245 Development of an osseous defect over a 3-month period. An acute abscess developed at this site but, as the symptoms abated, she did not seek professional advice. At her next routine visit it was found that a 9 mm pocket had developed on the mesial aspect of the first molar tooth. The tissue was red and oedematous with bleeding on minimal trauma. A new radiograph revealed a further 4 mm loss of bone.

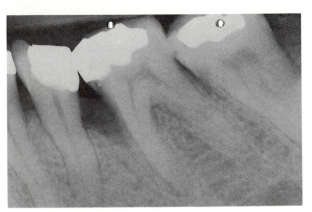

246 Repair after periodontal surgery. Periodontal surgery was performed using inverse bevel incisions, chronic inflammatory tissue being removed from the defect by curettage. Root planing of the cementum was carried out to the level of the previously determined base of pocket, avoiding excessive trauma to the deeper tissue, and the flaps sutured. Subsequently, there has been good repair of bone as indicated on the radiograph. Clinically there is 2 mm sulcus depth.

When there has been recent bone loss as a result of acute inflammation, several authors have advocated early surgical intervention. At this stage in the development of the acute lesion destruction is limited. The formation of an epithelial lining may be incomplete and there may still be residual collagen bundles.[2,3]

REPAIR OF A CHRONIC LESION, TREATED SURGICALLY

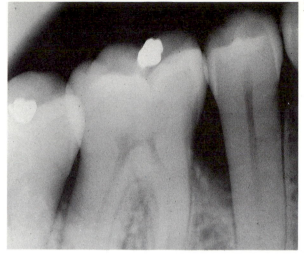

247 Radiograph of bone defect on the second premolar tooth. The radiograph shows a bone defect on the mandibular second premolar. The patient had completed the plaque control and root planing phase of treatment with minimal changes in the radiographic appearance.

248 (a) Diagram of the defect and (b) surgical treatment. Conservative inverse bevel incisions were used to raise buccal and lingual flaps. The epithelial lining and chronic inflammatory tissue were removed from the defect by curettage, and the root surfaces were planed to remove contaminants. The flaps were replaced with interrupted sutures, the objective being to achieve a good seal across the interproximal space, and so retain the blood clot.

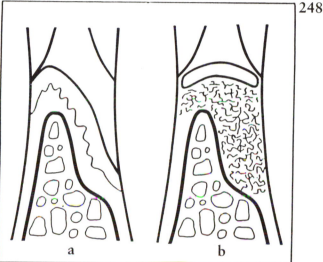

248

249 Bone defect after repair. This radiograph was taken 15 years after the one shown in **247**. There has been good repair of bone and this has remained stable throughout the maintenance phase of treatment. Repair of bone defects is not predictable. The degree of new bone formation depends on the type of bone defect, a narrow defect with 3 or 2 bony walls having the best prognosis.[4]

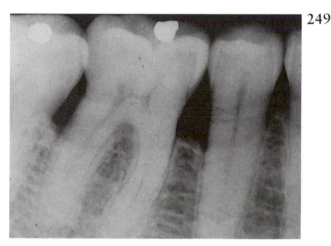

249

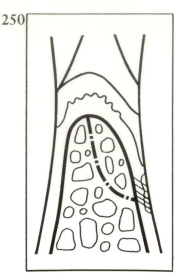

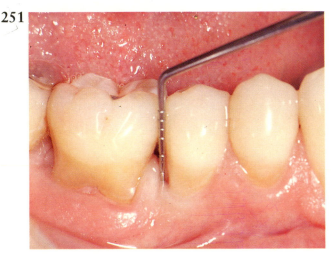

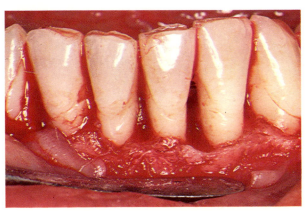

250 **The healing of bone defects.** The healing of bone defects treated by conservative surgical procedures has been reported in several studies.[5,6,7] It has been found that there is only a limited potential for new attachment of periodontal ligament fibres in bone defects (i.e. the formation of new connective tissue attachment and new cementum on root planed surface, previously contaminated). New attachment is restricted to a zone near the base of the bone defect extending 0.5 to 1 mm from the unaffected cementum. The source of the periodontal tissue comprising the new attachment is proliferation of cells from the periodontal ligament.[7]

Histological studies into the surgical treatment of bone defects that have 'filled in' have shown that there is a thin lining of junctional epithelium, often only a few cells thick, between the new bone and the previously affected cementum. This epithelium extends to within about 1 mm of the base of the previous defect;[5] however, this long junctional epithelial attachment does not seem to jeopardise the success of treatment.[8,9]

251 **Clinical result—minimal pocket depth** (see radiographs **247** and **249**). One of the most important factors influencing repair is the quality of plaque control. This patient had an excellent, indeed, almost over-enthusiastic preventive record as can be seen by the polished surfaces cervically. Fifteen years after treatment there is 2 mm sulcus depth at the site of the previous defect.

SURGICAL ELIMINATION OF OSSEOUS DEFECTS

252 **Osseous surgery in the mandibular anterior segment.** This patient has interproximal cratering and there is reverse architecture, the marginal bone being at a more coronal level than the interproximal bone. The marginal ledges are to be reduced and grooves established interproximally; this should be carried out very conservatively to restrict the removal of supporting bone.

253 Bone chisels being used to perform osseous surgery. A small amount of labial and lingual marginal bone is being removed to eliminate the craters and reduce the degree of reverse architecture. Bone chisels for periodontal surgery are available in various designs; there are angled ones for use in the posterior segments and finer-bladed instruments for interproximal regions. The one shown is from the Ochsenbein range. Alternatively, bone surgery may be carried out using a bur in a handpiece with a saline cooling spray.

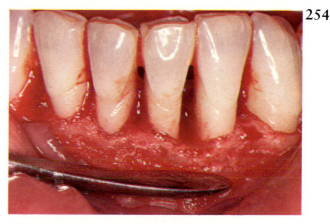

253

254 Assessing the contour after osseous surgery. Bone removal has been performed conservatively. It is inevitable that the raising of a flap and the cutting of bone will result in surgical trauma to the bone, with subsequent resorption and a further loss of about 0.5 to 1.0 mm of marginal bone during healing. This should be allowed for when undertaking osseous surgery.[10,11]

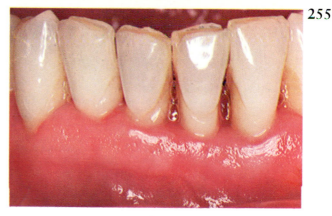

254

255 Clinical result. At 8 weeks after surgery there is no pocketing present. The conservative use of bone surgery on this patient, however, has resulted in a lack of scalloping in the gingival contour and a blunting of the interproximal papillae. This does not pose a hygiene problem to the well-motivated patient, and the acceptance of this type of contour is recommended in preference to the use of more radical ostectomy.

255

REPAIR USING GRAFTS AND IMPLANTS

A wide variety of materials has been used to occlude bone defects or to enhance the degree of regeneration. These include autografts of bone from oral sites,[12,13] frozen autograft from the iliac crest[14] or allografts, which have been treated, for example, by decalcification and freeze drying.[15] The disadvantages of these materials include problems with availability (in the case of autografts) and possible antigenicity (in the case of allografts).

More recently, the use of bone substitutes has received renewed attention. Most of these are derivatives of hydroxyapatite or tricalcium phosphate; both resorbable and non-resorbable forms have been used. Histological assessments in the early stages of healing have shown that, to a varying degree depending on their nature, the implants remain as inert granules surrounded by fibrous tissue. Some of the later assessments of the implanted material, however, show that after about 12 months there is evidence of new bone formation in juxtaposition to the hydroxyapatite crystals.[16]

With either natural bone or synthetic substitutes, there is no evidence of a greater degree of new attachment than with conventional procedures: long junctional epithelium being found between the graft/implant and cementum. Clinically in the case of deeper defects it has been found that postoperatively the depths of pockets are reduced and that the clinical attachment levels are located more coronally. Radiographically the material is shown to be well retained.[17,18,19]

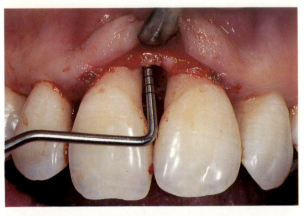

256 **Bone defect of 7 mm at time of surgery.** This patient had a deep infra-bony pocket between the central incisors and it was decided to use an implant to avoid the aesthetic disadvantages of osseous surgery. Intrasulcular incisions were used to retain the maximum amount of soft tissue and provide coverage of the implant subsequently. After the flap was raised, residual epithelial lining on the flap was removed and the papillae thinned. The infra-bony defect was curetted.

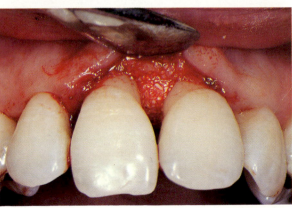

257 **Implant in the bone defect.** The defect has been filled with a non-resorbable hydroxyapatite implant. The crystals were placed into the defect incrementally and gently pressed into the confines of the defect so that they merged with the forming blood clot. The implant should not be built up excessively beyond the level of the existing bone.

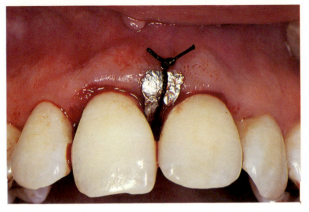

258 **The surgical site after suturing.** The flaps were brought together over the wound as closely as possible. In this case the seal over the interproximal region has been enhanced by means of adhesive tin foil, which was sutured in place.

259 Ten weeks after surgery. Preliminary healing had been uneventful and at 1 week the sutures were removed. Chlorhexidine mouthwash was used for 2 weeks after surgery. The patient has been on 3-weekly plaque control visits. Probing was carried out for the first time at this visit. It was found that there was resolution of the pocket and after probing there was no bleeding. Reduction of mobility is often a beneficial occurrence with this technique.

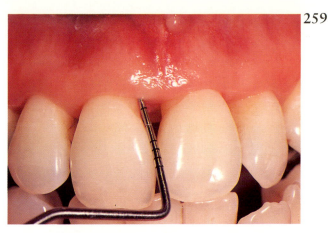
259

260 Pre-operative radiograph (left) compared with post-operative (right). The pre-operative radiographs show a deep osseous defect on the mesial side of the maxillary right incisor tooth. The post-operative radiograph which was taken at 6 months shows that the implanted hydroxyapatite has been retained well.

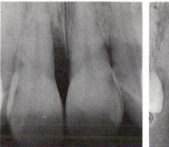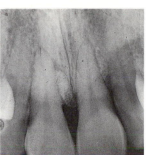
260

261 Histological appearance of an implant at 80 weeks (a) resorption; (b) deposition. This specimen was taken from a 49-year-old male patient. An infra-bony defect had been treated 80 weeks previously using a hydroxyapatite implant. It was decided to extract the tooth as it was still excessively mobile and interfering with function. A specimen to include the implant was removed surgically with the tooth. In general there was an absence of inflammatory cells around the implant. (a) In this section the dominant features were the spaces representing the implant particles surrounded by fibrous tissue. There were localised sites of resorption on the periphery of the particles. (b) At another site on the same specimen there was evidence of osteoid material being formed on the implanted material.

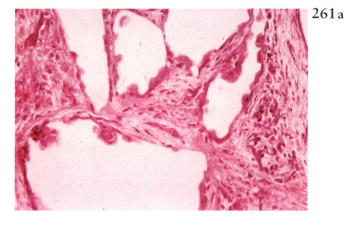
261a

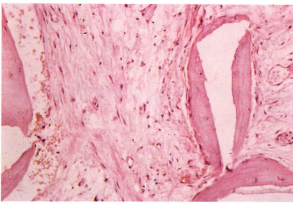
261b

When epithelium is injured there is a rapid system of repair, epithelial cells migrating from the uninjured margins of the wound as a result of increase in the rate of cell production. This cell migration is controlled by contact phenomena, for example, contact with connective tissue cells halts the advance of epithelial cells. The rate of epithelial cell turnover is controlled by mitotic inhibitors termed chalones.

Current research is investigating the use of various materials to guide the paths of epithelial cell proliferation, and to prevent their ingress into sites where it is desired to achieve regeneration of the periodontal tissues. Shielding the surgically prepared site from the ingress of epithelial cells enables periodontal tissue cells to proliferate in the area, and these cells have been shown to have the potential to form new periodontal ligament fibres which become inserted into bone and cementum.

262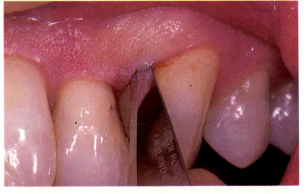

262 Pre-operative probing showing 7 mm pocket. After a prolonged course of periodontal treatment, including surgery in the posterior segments, the patient has a residual pocket on the distal aspect of the maxillary left lateral incisor. The treatment at this site has been restricted as the patient was anxious to avoid any recession. After being fully informed, the patient agreed to a guided tissue regeneration procedure being carried out at the site.

263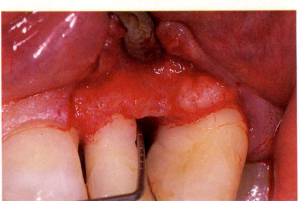

263 Conservative inverse bevel incision. A conservative incision is being used to preserve the existing gingival tissue for this procedure, as obtaining good wound closure is essential. Initially, the flap was restricted to the papilla between the incisor and canine teeth to enable the defect to be assessed. The flap was then developed to involve the neighbouring teeth subsequently. A relieving incision is recommended to aid access.

264

264 Bone defect 6 mm in depth. After reflection of the flap, granulation tissue was removed from the bone defect by curettage. Meticulous root planing with sharpened curettes was performed, and the site was then rinsed with saline to remove debris. A probe demonstrates the presence of a bone defect 6 mm in depth.

265 Membrane material trimmed to shape. The procedures for guided tissue regeneration were carried out according to the current methods recommended by the developers of the technique[20,21,22] and the manufacturer of the periodontal material. A template was first cut to fit around the cervical margins of the teeth and to overlap the margins of the bone defects by about 3 mm. This shape was then cut from the material. The curved collar of open-pore material, which is a feature of the design of the membrane, was left uncut and it was arranged that this collar would be applied to the lateral incisor tooth where the bone defect was deepest. The corners of the material were rounded to avoid subsequent perforation of the overlying flap.

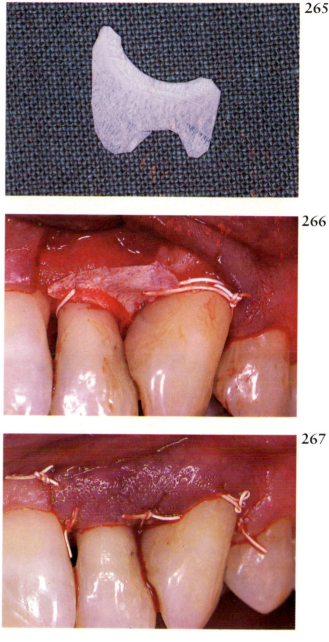

265

266

267

266 Membrane material sutured over the bone defect. The membrane material has been sutured in place by sling sutures around the involved teeth. It is important to avoid contamination of the membrane with saliva or by contact with gloves, so forceps were used to hold the material when cutting and suturing it. The open-pore collar can be seen to be enhancing the retention of a blood clot around the distal circumference of the lateral incisor tooth.

The rapid incorporation of fibrin and connective tissue in the porosity of the collar provides a circumferential seal, inhibiting the migration of epithelial cells apically as a result of contact inhibition. The smaller pores of the remainder of the membrane act as a mechanical barrier to the migration of epithelial cells.

267 Flap sutured in place. The flap was replaced and initially secured with interrupted sutures to achieve as good an interproximal seal as possible. The relieving incision was then sutured. Total coverage of the material by the flap has been recommended as it makes plaque removal easier.

No dressing was used after the procedure. The treated area was kept clean with chlorhexidine mouthwashes and the patient cautioned not to use floss in the surgical area. The sutures were removed after 1 week. During the following 8 weeks the patient was seen at fortnightly intervals.

268 Treated bone defect after removal of the membrane. Under local analgesia a secondary surgical procedure was undertaken. Flaps were raised and the membrane material removed. The bone defect had healed with newly regenerated tissue which was neither probed nor traumatised during this early stage in healing. The inner aspects of the flaps were curetted to remove epithelium and then replaced and secured with interrupted sutures which were removed a week later.

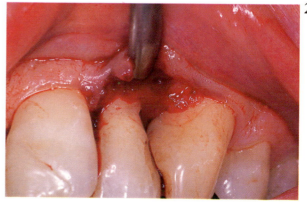

268

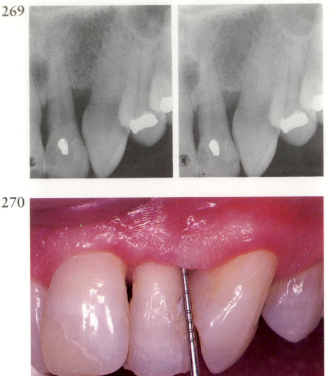

269 Pre-operative and 4 months post-operative radiographs. The degree of bone formation currently reported with the use of guided tissue regeneration techniques is variable. These radiographs indicate that there may have been slight increase in bone density in the deepest portion of the treated defect. Future developments may involve combined guidance of soft tissue healing with techniques for enhanced induction of bone formation.

270 Clinical healing at 4 months. On the lateral incisor tooth there is now a healthy periodontal condition, with 2 mm sulcus depth and no bleeding on probing.

Further research is necessary to achieve an easily applied, effective membrane system for the prevention of the ingress of epithelium; more knowledge is required about the ideal chemical and physical properties for this type of membrane. It would be desirable to develop a biodegradable material, obviating the need for a secondary surgical procedure.[23]

SUMMARY

There is continuing research into techniques for the treatment of periodontal bone defects, with the emphasis on achieving regeneration or repair of the lost periodontal tissues.[24] The selection of a technique should be based on the principle of conserving bone even if, occasionally, a further re-entry procedure may be necessary to modify the bone contour after only partial success with a conservative surgical procedure.

14 INTER-RELATED PERIODONTAL AND ENDODONTIC LESIONS, AND FURCATION INVOLVEMENT

The inter-relationship between periodontal and endodontic lesions can be represented diagrammatically:[1]

PRIMARY
ENDODONTIC LESION

↓

SECONDARY PERIODONTAL
INVOLVEMENT

PRIMARY
PERIODONTAL LESION

↓

SECONDARY ENDODONTIC
INVOLVEMENT

INDEPENDENT CO-EXISTENT
PATHOLOGY

↓

COMBINED LESION

It is important to diagnose the primary causes of inter-related periodontal and endodontic lesions, as the treatment plan is subsequently based on this knowledge.[2] The various tests that should be undertaken have been described (see 83 to 87), and their interpretation will usually determine the aetiology of the condition.

PRIMARY ENDODONTIC LESION WITH SECONDARY PERIODONTAL INVOLVEMENT

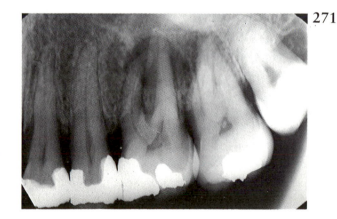

271

271 Radiograph showing radiolucencies in the periapical and trifurcation regions. The upper left first molar tooth has a periapical radiolucency which extends into the trifurcation of the roots. There is an associated abscess discharging via the periodontal ligament into the trifurcation, and from there into the gingival sulcus buccally. When tested, the pulp was non-vital.

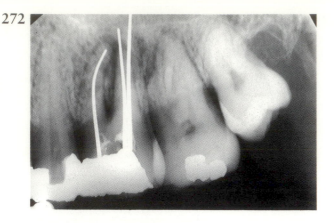

272 After endodontic treatment. The primary cause of the lesion was treated and endodontic therapy carried out on the upper first molar tooth. The furcation region should be gently cleaned of debris, plaque being removed with a curette using light pressure. The use of chlorhexidine solution in a syringe to irrigate sub-gingivally may be beneficial.

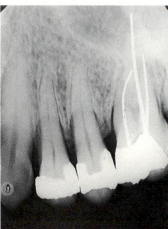

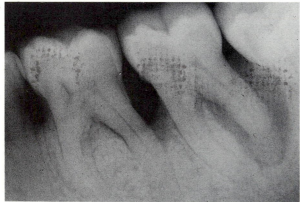

273 Six months after root treatment. The patient has been on a regular periodontal maintenance programme. Six months after the endodontic treatment, the rarefaction both in the apical regions and in the trifurcation has resolved. The opening to the furcations could no longer be probed from any aspect of the tooth.

In the longer standing endodontic-periodontal lesion, the communication into the gingival sulcus may become epithelialised, in which event a sinus tract may persist after endodontic treatment. This epithelial lining would be removed surgically.

PRIMARY PERIODONTAL LESION WITH SECONDARY ENDODONTIC INVOLVEMENT

274 Primary periodontal lesion with secondary endodontic involvement. The patient has a generalised periodontitis; the lower second molar tooth had a severe degree of periodontal involvement on the distal root extending beyond the apex. When tested, the pulp of this tooth was found to be non-vital. As the primary lesion was periodontal, the main emphasis was on this aspect of treatment, the aim being to ensure that the periodontitis in other areas of the mouth was controlled.

It is usually necessary to treat both the periodontal and endodontic conditions, although periodontal lesions with associated periapical problems have been reported in which the periapical radiolucency resolved following periodontal treatment alone.[3]

INDEPENDENT CO-EXISTENT PERIODONTAL AND ENDODONTIC LESIONS

The patient shown (369 to 378) had residual periodontal pockets after a preventive programme. There were also co-existent periapical radiolucencies. It is often of benefit to combine the necessary surgical procedures so that the two separate types of lesion, although independent, are treated together. The basis for being able to integrate treatment in this way is a thorough diagnosis.

COMBINED PERIODONTAL AND ENDODONTIC LESION

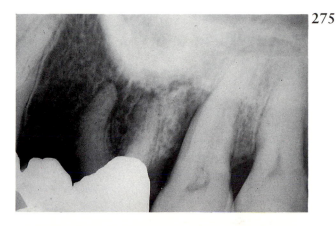

275

275   Recently constructed bridge—periapical radiolucencies. This referred patient recently had a bridge constructed on the first molar tooth and was now complaining of palatal swelling in this region. The radiograph revealed periapical radiolucencies. Unfortunately, there had been no consideration of endodontic treatment or periodontal treatment before the placement of the bridge.

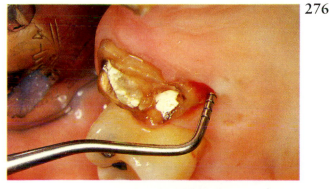

276

276   Periodontal assessment after removal of the bridge. The bridge was removed to aid access for treatment and periodontal probing revealed a 9 mm pocket involving the palatal root. The disto-palatal furcation was also involved; it was unclear whether this involvement was primarily of periodontal or endodontic origin or from both, as seemed more probable. The endodontic lesions on the distal or palatal roots may have been discharging via the periodontal ligament or via an accessory root canal into the furcation region.

277   After endodontic and periodontal treatment. The buccal roots of the upper first molar tooth and the two roots on the upper first premolar tooth, which were also non-vital, have been endodontically treated. The crown of the molar was then sectioned and the palatal root extracted, leaving the buccal roots. A new bridge has been constructed, and the patient is symptom-free.

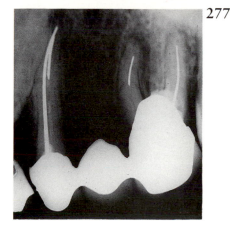

277

SUMMARY

The correct diagnosis of inter-related periodontal endodontic lesions is crucial to the success of treatment. The primary cause of the lesion is usually treated first. The order of treatment is especially important in the case of a lesion with primarily endodontic involvement, as root treatment alone will often result in complete resolution.

The treatment of furcation problems

On a multi-rooted tooth the furcation region is where the main body of the root divides to form the several components. When bone loss and apical migration of the junctional epithelium exposes the furcation to the oral environment, problems in treatment arise as a result of the complex morphology of the inter-radicular region, which interferes with access for the removal of plaque and calculus deposits by both patient and clinician. A number of factors influence the stage in development of periodontitis at which furcation involvement becomes a problem. Some of the most important factors are morphological considerations, such as the distance of the opening of the furcations from the enamel-cement junction, the contour of the roots, the presence of enamel projections extending towards the furcation region, and the contour of the overlying alveolar bone.[4,5,6] Several systems have been devised for classifying furcation involvement; the ideal system should take account of both the horizontal and vertical extent of the involvement.[7] The horizontal involvement may either be measured with a probe and recorded in millimetres, or may be classified as:

Grade 1, where there is incipient involvement in which just the opening of the furcation is exposed.
Grade II, where the involvement extends into or beyond the central portion of the furcation.
Grade III, through and through involvement.

The vertical component of involvement can best be expressed in millimetres measured from the commencement of the furcation to the base of the bone defect.

The treatment of a tooth with furcation involvement depends on:

1   The degree of bone loss involving the various roots.
2   The morphology of the bone defect.
3   The contour of the furcation walls.
4   The shape of the roots.
5   The relationship with neighbouring teeth.
6   The restorative and endodontic condition of the tooth.

A key factor in deciding treatment is the overall treatment plan for the patient, the management of localised complex problems clearly having to be integrated with treatment procedures in the other areas of the mouth.

CONSERVATIVE TREATMENT

The treatment of Class I furcation lesions is usually restricted to procedures making the region more easily cleanable by the patient. Minor modifications to the contour of the soft tissue to correct pockets may be indicated. It may be helpful to recontour the region on the tooth near the opening to the furcation, by widening-out narrow fissure-like openings to aid access for cleaning.[8] More severely involved teeth may also be treated conservatively but adequate access for instrumentation in the furcation is often difficult (see **278**). Although the results cannot be predicted accurately, a proportion of teeth with furcation involvement, treated relatively conservatively by plaque control and root planing, including flap surgery if necessary, may be retained for many years.[9,10] In one study, teeth treated in this way were followed for periods from 5 to 24 years, 88 per cent being retained throughout the study.[9]

Newer treatment techniques for furcation involvement are being introduced that include the principles of guided tissue regeneration and techniques for enhancing the compatibility of the root surface for new attachment.[11,12]

TECHNIQUES TO ENHANCE ACCESS FOR CLEANING PROCEDURES

The conservative management of a tooth with furcation involvement results in an uncertain prognosis. More definitive procedures should be considered, where a more predictable outcome is required; for example, when the tooth is of key importance in the general treatment plan, or where there is a danger of interproximal bone loss associated with a furcation involving the septum shared with a healthy tooth. Such techniques include tunnel procedures, root amputation or sectioning of the tooth. There may also be the need for associated endodontic and restorative treatment.[13,14,15,16] The extraction of the tooth should always be considered as an option where the tooth is not an important one or where it can be incorporated in a prosthetic treatment plan (see **282** and **283**).

DIAGNOSIS

The treatment plan must be based on a correct assessment and diagnosis. Investigations should include pocket depth measurements, probing of the furcation region from all aspects, radiographs and vitality tests. Assessment of the endodontic status of teeth with furcation involvement is of particular importance, as it is necessary that teeth with joint pathology be diagnosed and the appropriate treatment instigated for both components (see **271** to **277**).

278 Extracted tooth demonstrating restricted access to furcation. The very narrow apertures between the roots of some teeth with furcation involvement make access for removal of deposits almost impossible. Even the finest periodontal instruments are too large to gain entry to a considerable proportion of furcation regions.[17]

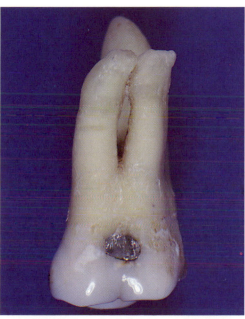

278

279 Extracted tooth demonstrating concave surfaces of walls and roof of furcation region. Removal of plaque and calculus from the furcation region is also hindered by the concave contour of the root surfaces that form the furcation walls, and by the dome shape and the ridges frequently found in the roof of the furcation.[18,19]

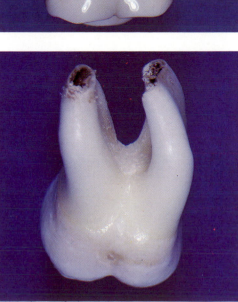

279

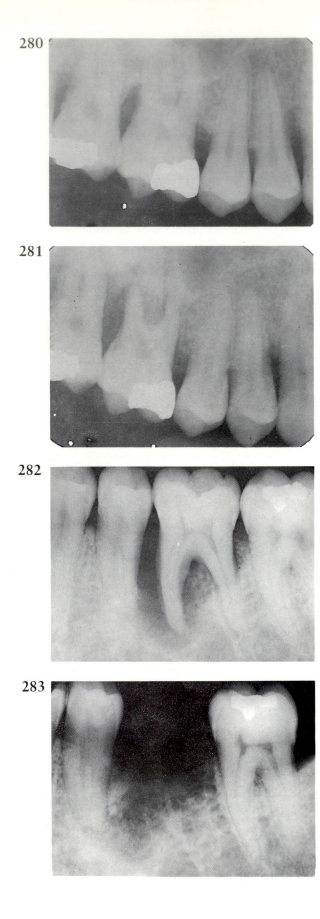

280   **Maxillary molar teeth with Grade III furcation involvement.** The patient, a 43-year-old man, received periodontal treatment comprising plaque control and root planing for all his dentition. Particular care was taken in treating the furcation regions of the maxillary molar teeth as there was Grade III furcation involvement on these teeth. He was advised that there was a poor prognosis for the molar teeth without undergoing more complex procedures. After a thorough discussion about the various alternatives, he declined to have surgical treatment but wished to retain the teeth for as long as possible. The maintenance programme involved 3-monthly visits for plaque control, with particular attention being paid to the thorough removal of deposits from the residual pockets on the molar teeth. The ultrasonic scaler is very helpful for debridement in furcation regions.[20]

281   **Radiograph taken 10 years later.** The radiograph shows that there has been further loss of bone in the furcation regions but the teeth were still functional. Teeth with furcation involvement can be treated conservatively and, although the long-term prognosis is uncertain, a considerable period of satisfactory function can often be achieved.

THE ROLE OF EXTRACTION

282   **Severe bone loss and furcation involvement.** When there is uneven severe bone loss affecting one or more teeth and, particularly, when the shared interproximal septum of a sound tooth is being involved by periodontal disease on an adjacent tooth, then extraction may be the treatment of choice. It was decided to extract this mandibular left first molar tooth.

283   **Bone deposition in socket 1 year later.** The radiograph taken 1 year later shows that bone has been deposited in the socket. The prognosis of the second premolar tooth has been greatly improved and the patient is now being assessed with a view to the provision of a fixed prosthesis.

OPERATIVE PROCEDURES SPECIFICALLY FOR MULTIROOTED TEETH

The tunnel procedure

284 Mandibular molar tooth to be treated by tunnel procedure. When a tooth with bifurcation involvement has a wide U-shaped arch between the roots, this may be opened out surgically with osteoplasty and odontoplasty. The soft tissue contour is also adapted to achieve good access for subsequent cleaning.

285 Access for cleaning demonstrated. After treatment by the tunnel procedure, the patient must be given special instruction in cleaning the bifurcation region. An interdental brush may be the best implement for plaque removal from the furcation, as the walls and roof are usually concave in shape. The use of fluoride gel on the brush is beneficial as caries tends to be a problem in the bifurcation after this procedure.[13]

Root amputation

286 Pre-operative condition—furcation involvement. On the mandibular left first molar tooth there is a 10 mm pocket on the distal root with an associated infra-bony defect involving the bifurcation. There is minimal bone loss on the mesial root of this tooth. Vital extirpation of the pulp was carried out, the mesial root canals being permanently root-filled, whereas the distal root canal was occluded with calcium hydroxide paste as a temporary measure. It is preferable to carry out pulp extirpation before amputating roots. Although the pulp of a vital tooth which has been treated by root amputation can be covered with a dressing at the time of surgery, the resultant hyperaemia can cause problems in achieving analgesia for subsequent extirpation.

287 Radiograph after amputation of the distal root. The distal root of the tooth has been amputated. After extraction of the root the bone margins were smoothed, the root surfaces were planed and chronic inflammatory tissue and pocket lining removed from the flaps of soft tissue around the socket. The flaps were closed with sutures after completion of these procedures. In this case, the crown of the tooth was left intact to act as a temporary space maintainer while the socket healed. Judicious occlusion adjustment may be used to reduce occlusal loads on the unsupported portion of the crown.

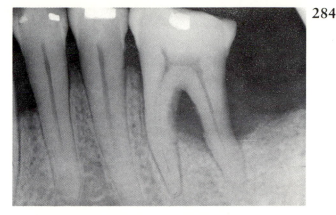

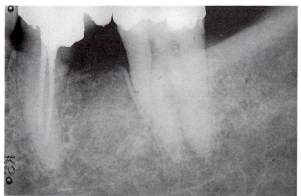

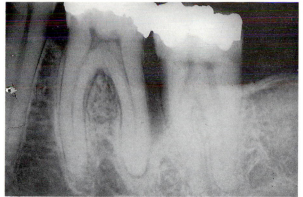

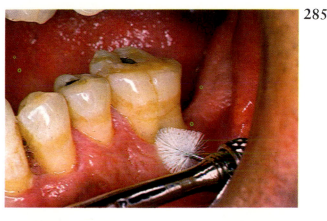

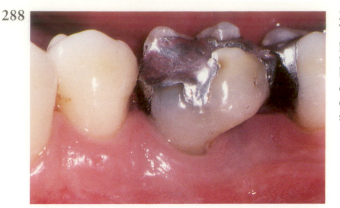

288 The clinical condition 3 months after surgery.
The soft tissue contour is now satisfactory, with no pocketing around the mesial root of the first molar tooth. Modification of cleaning procedures has been demonstrated, the techniques involving the careful use of floss to clean under the distal cantilever of the crown, especially at the previous site of the bifurcation.

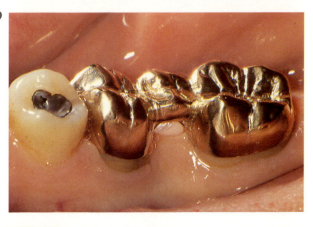

289 Restoration with a bridge. There is a danger that the weakened crown of a tooth may fracture after root amputation, with the possibility of the fracture line extending subgingivally, sometimes even necessitating extraction of the tooth. For this reason, once the prognosis for the tooth has been established, a more permanent restoration should be undertaken.[21]

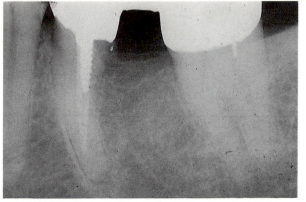

290 Radiograph to show bone deposition in socket. Six months after surgery, new bone has been deposited within the socket and the roots of both the neighbouring teeth have good bone contour.

  The use of root amputation for palatal root involvement on an upper molar tooth has been described (see **275** to **277**).

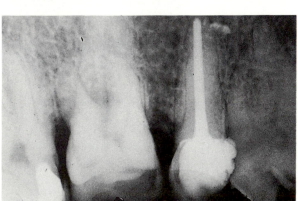

291 Maxillary tooth with severely involved disto-buccal root. This maxillary upper first molar tooth has severe bone loss on the disto-buccal root. Of the 3 roots on an upper molar tooth, this root generally has the smallest surface area,[22] hence its amputation has only a minimal effect on the remaining tooth support.

292   Clinical result 2 years after root amputation.
The follow-up after the amputation of the
disto-buccal root shows a satisfactory result. The
relatively large embrasure opening requires the
continuing use of either a single-tufted or
interdental brush (see **148** and **156**).

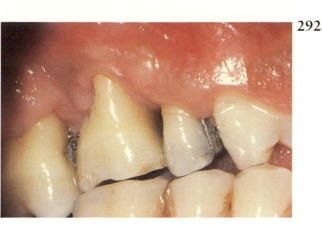

292

293   After disto-buccal root amputation. Two
years after root amputation, the socket has healed
well with minimal pocketing or bone defects on the
remaining roots. It was considered unnecessary to
restore the crown of this tooth as the distal structure
was sound and there was adequate strength to resist
fracture.

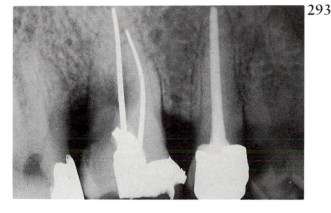

293

294   Incorrect technique for root amputation. The
mesio-buccal root of this maxillary first molar was
treated by attempted root amputation. The
procedure was inadequately performed, and a
spur-shaped fragment of root is still present
adjoining the furcation region. When carrying out
root amputation, the sectioning of the root should
commence with the bur placed in the furcation. The
cut is then made towards the interproximal cervical
margin so that a smooth line of emergence is
achieved. If the furcation is too narrow to permit
entry for the bur, access is gained by cutting into the
root to be removed thus creating, within the
furcation, a clear starting point for the procedure.

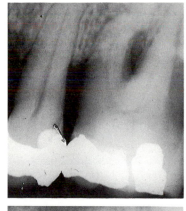

294a

294b

295

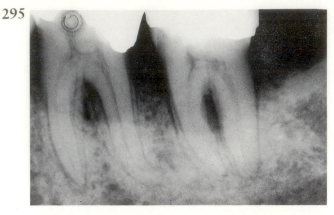

295   First and second molar teeth—furcation involvement. The second molar tooth has no opposing unit and it is proposed to extract it. The first molar tooth has relatively widely spaced roots and it has been decided to section the tooth and restore it as 2 units, enabling access to be gained to the present furcation region for cleaning by routine use of dental floss.

296

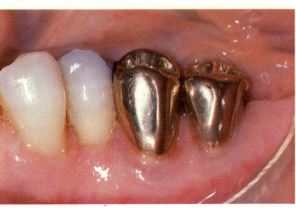

296   Clinical appearance after sectioning and restoration. Six years after surgery, the restored units are associated with a healthy gingival condition. The patient has, in effect, 4 premolar teeth and can clean the interproximal areas without recourse to special aids.

297

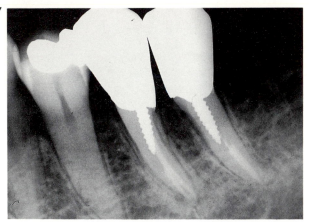

297   Radiograph 6 years after sectioning. The condition of the alveolar bone appears stable. It can be seen that the inter-radicular root space is restricted near the cervical margin. If the space had been any narrower, orthodontic treatment would have been necessary to move the roots further apart before restorative treatment.

CONCLUSION

Furcation lesions pose a unique problem in periodontal treatment because of the severely restricted access for treatment procedures and subsequent plaque control. Treatment options vary in complexity, ranging from conservative treatment involving the removal of all the accessible deposits and subsequent maintenance, to more comprehensive therapy involving endodontic and restorative procedures before surgical treatment, including amputation of one or more roots or sectioning of a tooth to enable access to be gained to the furcation for routine cleaning.

The width of attached gingiva varies considerably from individual to individual and tooth to tooth.[1] The width may be further influenced by the relative size of the teeth and jaws and by any anomaly in tooth alignment.

Inflammation, induced either by irritants from plaque or trauma to gingival tissue, may cause proliferation of epithelial cells into the connective tissue of the corium. The associated subsidence of the epithelial surface is manifested as gingival recession, with a reduction in the width of keratinised gingiva.[2]

Muco-gingival aberrations may cause aesthetic or functional problems.[3,4]

AESTHETIC PROBLEMS

While the implications of aesthetics are a very individual matter, in many cases localised or generalised recession, especially in the anterior maxillary region, may result in patients requesting corrective treatment. The long-term success of muco-gingival procedures in treating recession cannot be predicted with certainty, however, and patients should be so advised.

FUNCTIONAL PROBLEMS

From a functional point of view, the relationship between a reduction in the width of attached gingiva and periodontal health is somewhat controversial. There have been reports suggesting a need for a minimum 1mm width of attached gingiva if periodontal health is to be maintained.[5] Subsequent work has established that, with good plaque control, a healthy periodontal condition can coexist with neither gingivitis nor increased recession in the absence of a zone of attached gingiva.[6,7,8] If maintenance of plaque control is neglected, or if the concentration of irritants is increased, for example by placement of sub-gingival restorations, then inadequate widths of gingiva are associated, perhaps, with a greater degree of gingivitis.[9,10,11]

Frenal insertions are considered by some to be of aetiological significance if they exert a pull on the attached tissue, because they may cause recession of the gingival margin. Unfortunately, there are few longitudinal studies to support or refute this view and clinicians still have to use their clinical judgement to decide whether surgical treatment is appropriate.

Where there is midline spacing of the maxillary incisor teeth, the large fibres of the frenum have been found to cause disruption of the transeptal fibre system. Thus, frenectomy may be indicated as part of the treatment plan for orthodontic closure of the midline space.[12]

Frenectomy

Frenectomy is used mainly on the labial aspect of the upper and lower anterior regions but may also be used on the buccal segments and for the treatment of a lingual frenum. The objectives of the procedure are to eliminate a frenum and to create a zone of keratinised gingiva at the former site of insertion.

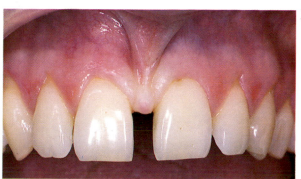

298

298   Pre-operative condition. This patient has completed a plaque control programme. The frenum is an impediment to good cleaning and as a result of the associated inflammation, the area between the central incisors still bleeds on probing. In addition, retraction of the lip tends to exert a pull on the gingival margin, possibly aiding plaque ingress to the gingival sulcus region.

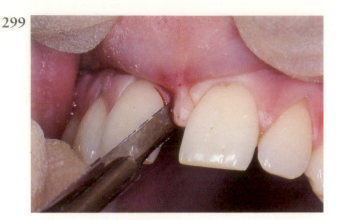

299 Incisions labially. With the lip retracted, an initial incision is made along the lateral border of the frenum, commencing at the muco-gingival junction and passing interdentally as far as the incisive papilla. A similar incision is made on the other side of the frenum. Every care must be taken to conserve all the keratinised gingival tissue.

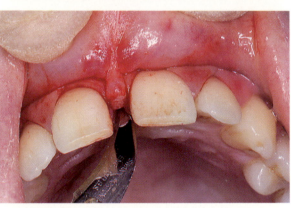

300 Incision palatally. A palatal transverse incision is made anterior to the incisive papilla, which joins up the previous incisions. A number 12 blade is being used.

301 Frenum reflected. The frenum is freed from the underlying bone either by sharp dissection to retain the periosteum, or by blunt dissection separating periosteum from bone with a periosteal elevator. The retention of periosteum will increase the rate of epithelialisation.

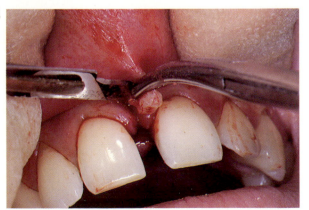

302 Excision of frenum. Using curved artery forceps, the frenum is now grasped and is dissected free from the mucosa of the labial aspect of the vestibule and then removed.

303 Suturing completed. The mucosa is sutured to approximate the edges of the wound. A diagonal suturing technique across the interproximal space was used.

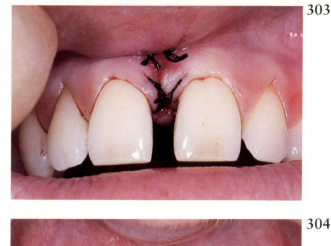

303

304 Postoperative result. As a result of the frenectomy, there is no longer interference with hygiene and there is no bleeding of the gingiva on probing. The patient is under review prior to the orthodontic closure of the midline space.

304

Gingival grafting procedures

The gingival graft procedure is used to increase locally the width of gingiva.[13,4] The relationship between gingival inflammation and the width of gingiva is controversial, as discussed earlier. Attempts should be made to control gingivitis by plaque control measures and only if these fail, or if gingival recession is progressing should gingival grafting be considered. The procedure is also used to correct recession but the result is not then entirely predictable, as it relies during initial healing on diffusion to achieve adequate nourishment to the grafted tissue bridging the previously exposed root surface.

It has been demonstrated by several workers that the stimuli causing epithelium to keratinise originate in the underlying connective tissue.[14,15] The principles of gingival grafting are based on the conservation and relocation of existing keratinised tissue, including the underlying corium, so that the resultant epithelium is induced to keratinise.

Gingival graft used to correct frenal problem

305 Pre-operative condition. The plaque control phase of treatment has been completed for this patient. There is recession and persistence of marginal inflammation on the mandibular left central incisor evidenced by localised bleeding on probing. This may be attributed to an absence of attached gingiva and an active labial frenum, causing retraction of the margin which aids the ingress of micro-organisms. The gingival graft procedure is to be used to increase the width of keratinised gingiva.

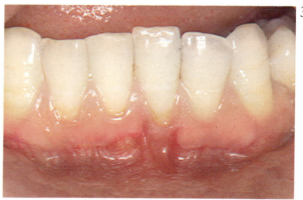

305

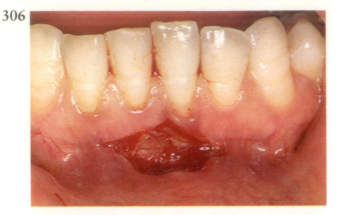

306 Graft bed prepared. An incision is made along the muco-gingival junction and sharp dissection is used to prepare the graft bed. The prognosis of the graft procedure is improved when a band of gingival tissue can be retained, thus creating a recipient site with a circumferential blood supply. The alveolar mucosa, muscle attachments and periosteum are displaced apically, exposing bone.[16,17,18] Where the area to be grafted is larger, and the attainment of a blood supply is a priority, periosteum may be retained over bone in the area to be grafted by using sharp dissection. It is important that the mucosal flap is made sufficiently mobile by dissection to prevent its subsequent encroachment on to the grafted area during healing.

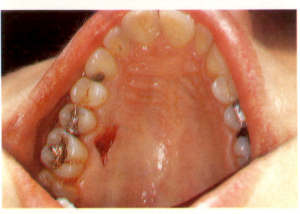

307 Donor site. An appropriate donor site is selected. The most common site is the keratinised tissue of the palate. The outline incision for the graft is made about 3 mm away from the gingival margin. Starting from the coronal edge a graft of about 1.5 mm thickness is prepared by dissection, which incorporates some of the corium from the donor site. Following the preparation of the graft, it should be transferred with as little delay as possible to the site to be grafted.

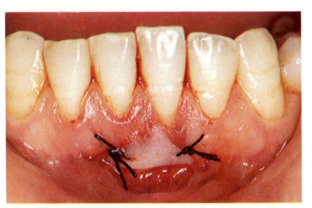

308 Graft maintenance. The graft is maintained in position by fine sutures (00000). These must not be placed under tension. Pressure is applied to the graft for 5 minutes to prevent the formation of a haematoma and to promote the formation of an initial fibrin attachment, with the graft and donor site in close proximity.[19] A dressing may be placed over the grafted area. At the donor site, retention of a dressing may prove difficult and a suture over the dressing may help. For larger donor areas, an acrylic palatal plate may be used to prevent the wound from being traumatised and to reduce pain.

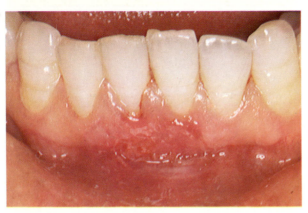

309 One week postoperative result. On removal of the dressing and sutures after 1 week, it can be seen that the superficial layers of epithelial cells have been shed from the grafted tissue. Attachment has been established between the corium of the graft and the recipient site. There is usually no need to apply another dressing. Instruction in postoperative oral hygiene is essential.

310 Eight weeks postoperative result. Eight weeks after surgery the grafted gingiva is paler than the surrounding tissue. This is often a permanent characteristic and may be caused by an increased thickness of either the keratinised epithelium or the corium. There is a firm attachment of the graft to underlying bone. The effectiveness of the graft procedure has been demonstrated,[20] and it was reported that the treatment of localised areas of recession resulted in a mean new junctional epithelium attachment of 1.1 mm, a reduction in pocketing of 0.4 mm and a reduction in recession of 0.7 mm. Although the gingival graft procedure has been shown to increase the zone of keratinised and attached gingiva, more recent studies have indicated that there is no influence on the amount of plaque or inflammation.[21,22]

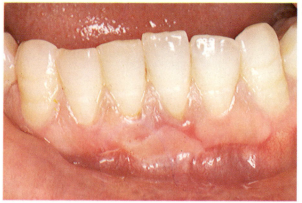

310

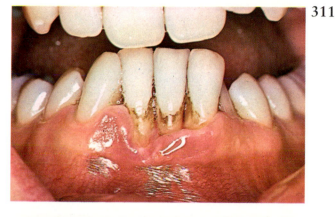

311

Gingival graft to resist functional trauma to soft tissues

311 Trauma to mandibular labial gingiva. The patient has an Angle Class II division ii malocclusion and the upper incisor teeth occlude on to the labial gingiva of the lower incisor teeth.

312 Gingival graft providing resistance to trauma. A gingival graft has been placed to achieve a zone of keratinised gingiva. The dense tissue of the graft was considered to provide better resistance to the traumatic functional forces of the opposing teeth.

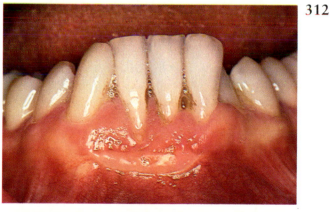

312

Gingival graft used to modify an edentulous ridge

313 Local pigmentation of the ridge. There is unsightly pigmentation of the ridge as a result of silver amalgam particles retained in the soft tissues after a previous attempt at a retrograde root treatment. A bridge is to be constructed to replace the missing maxillary anterior teeth.

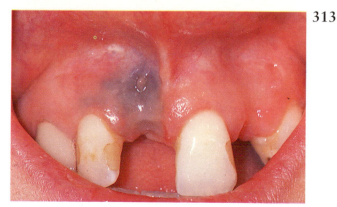

313

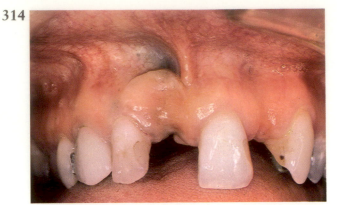

314

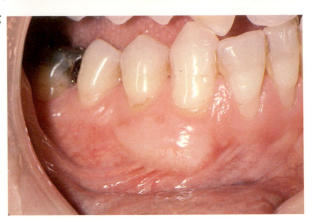

315

314 Graft replacing the discoloured soft tissue. A relatively thick graft was used to replace the discoloured tissue. Where there has been a degree of ridge resorption, the use of a graft with increased amount of corium may be used to correct the contour and improve aesthetics.[23]

Subepithelial connective tissue graft to correct recession

315 Gingival graft using corium only. Ten years previously, treatment had been carried out to correct progressive recession on the labial aspect of this mandibular canine tooth. A graft was used from the corium of the palatal tissue comprising connective tissue only.[24,4] Subsequent epithelialisation occurred from the peripheral tissue, and the principle of induction is illustrated by the graft becoming keratinised to form gingiva.

Areas of recession may be corrected using a gingival graft in this way (usually including epithelium as well as corium). The scope for success of this procedure is dependent on the potential for diffusion of nutrients to the graft from the margins of the wound. The blood supply can be enhanced by bevelling the wound edges to increase the surface area and by obtaining close adaption of the graft to the bed, using vertical or horizontal stay sutures over the graft (see **323**).

Laterally repositioned flap

The laterally repositioned flap can be used as an alternative to the free gingival graft to treat a localised muco-gingival defect. The survival of the transposed tissue is more predictable compared with a gingival graft as it has its own blood supply, which is of particular relevance when it is placed over an exposed root surface for the correction of recession. The prognosis is best when the recession is associated with a relatively narrow, shallow dehiscence and where there is minimal loss of interproximal bone on either side of the defect. In addition, there should be no dehiscence or fenestration of the alveolar plate on the donor tooth and, ideally, the donor gingiva should be relatively thick.[25]

316

316 Pre-operative condition. This patient is concerned about recession involving the mandibular central incisors. Following initial therapy, there is persistent gingivitis and also an aesthetic problem, as he shows the mandibular anterior gingiva when he speaks. Laterally repositioned flaps are to be used to treat the condition, in preference to a gingival graft, in view of the surface area of root to be covered.

317 Incisions. The marginal gingiva and sulcular epithelium are removed around the area of recession and the root surfaces planed to remove deposits and to reduce the root prominence.

The design of the flap for lateral repositioning is very important as there must be a compromise between the need to achieve an adequate width and thickness of gingival tissue on the flap, and the need to avoid recession at the donor site. At the donor site periosteum may be retained by using split thickness dissection, and a coronal band of marginal gingiva, about 1.5 mm in width, may also be retained to reduce the possibility of recession.[26] In this case, emphasis is on coverage of the root surface on the neighbouring teeth, hence no marginal gingiva has been retained at the donor site. Vertical incisions in the gingiva are made to delineate the extremities of the donor site near line angles, so that interproximal bone will be exposed when the flap is transposed, rather than marginal bone which is thinner.

318 Flaps laterally positioned. Sufficient mobility of the tissues must be achieved by dissection to enable the flaps to be moved to the new sites without any tension. Mobility can be enhanced by the design of the initial incisions, these being angled so that the base of the flap is biased towards the direction in which the flap is to be moved.

319 Modification of procedure, grafts on donor sites. As an adjunct to healing and to reduce the possibility of recession, in this case, gingival grafts have been placed at the donor sites. This modification enables the emphasis to be placed on achieving adequate tissue to make up the flaps, without concern about retaining tissue at the donor sites.[27] The alternative, conventional procedure is to leave the donor site to heal by epithelialisation from the surrounding tissue. Fine sutures (00000) are used to avoid damaging the relatively fragile tissues.

320 Postoperative condition. The tissues have healed well and the amount of recession has been reduced on the central incisors; the sulcus on these teeth is about 1.5 mm deep. Recession on the donor teeth has been avoided by using gingival grafts. Histological studies have shown that the new attachment of the gingiva to the recipient tooth is achieved by cementogenesis and new connective tissue attachment in the apical zone, and by the attachment of junctional epithelium to the tooth more coronally.[28]

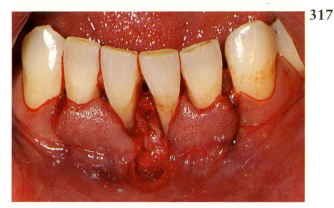

317

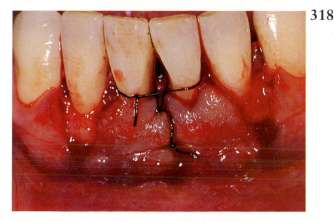

318

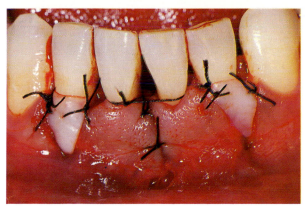

319

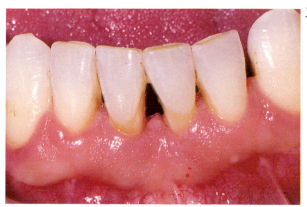

320

Other types of pedicle flap procedure

Several other types of pedicle flap procedure have been described and there may be occasions when the tissue configuration favours their application. For example, the double papillae flap involves raising the papillae adjoining the area of marginal recession.[29] The papillae are moved across as pedicle flaps and the freshly bevelled edges are sutured together. The disadvantage is that the suture line lies over the root surface to be covered and may break down during healing or may be a subsequent zone of weakness. The coronally repositioned graft is another alternative.

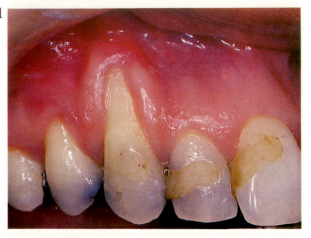

321 Coronally repositioned gingival graft. The success of treating localised gingival recession depends on the size of the area of recession and the choice of procedure depends on the availability of donor tissue. Where there is a problem in finding a source of tissue locally, or where it is essential to avoid causing recession on neighbouring teeth, the coronally repositioned gingival graft may be considered.[30,31] This is a two-stage procedure in which tissue of sufficient size and thickness is first grafted in place and, subsequently, when a good vascular supply has been established, it is moved coronally.

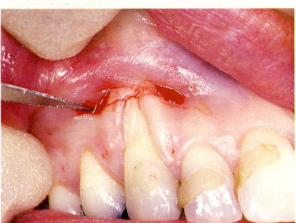

322 Incision for the preparation of the graft bed. A horizontal incision through to bone is made at the level of the gingival recession. A periosteal elevator is then used to reflect soft tissue and prepare the site on which the gingival graft is to be placed.

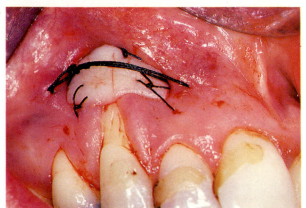

323 Gingival graft sutured in place. A gingival graft was taken from the palatal donor site. The size of the graft should be larger than the size of the defect to allow for a degree of shrinkage. It has been sutured in place and a horizontal stay suture has been placed to apply pressure.

324　Healed graft after 2 months. The sutures were removed after 1 week. This shows the condition after 2 months.

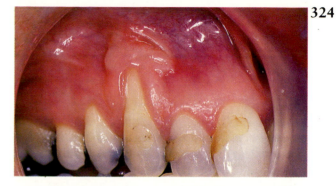

324

325　Incisions for coronal repositioning. Two vertical incisions are made, starting in the vestibule and extending to the tooth. These permit the graft to be freed from the underlying bone. The incisions are placed over bone and are designed to achieve an adequate blood supply to the wound.

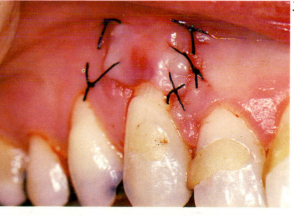

325

326　Coronal repositioning of graft. The flap containing the graft is coronally repositioned and sutured in place. It is important that the wound edges are closely approximated to achieve primary healing.

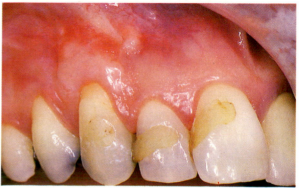

326

327　Postoperative result 3 months after coronal repositioning. The sutures were removed after 1 week; this shows the situation 3 months later. While this procedure can produce excellent results, some recurrence of recession may be anticipated and the patient should be warned accordingly.

327

16 RELATIONSHIP BETWEEN OCCLUSION AND PERIODONTAL DISEASE

For many years there has been debate concerning possible association between periodontal disease and occlusal trauma. The basis for such a hypothesis may have been that symptoms, such as changes in alveolar bone density, increase in tooth mobility and migration of teeth, were shared by both phenomena. The experimental work investigating occlusion and periodontal disease has been based on post-mortem interpretation of human autopsy material and on carefully designed animal studies. Recent work has produced many useful results, although some doubt inevitably will remain about the interpretation of animal research. Clinical studies are hindered by ethical problems in carrying out experimental procedures involving irreversible changes in humans.

The work reported in the following review has been carried out in monkeys, with application of mesial and distal alternating forces applied by interproximal wedges changed every 48 hours. Other work has used dogs, with forces being applied by means of combined occlusal ramps and counteracting springs. Where differences between results have occurred, it is difficult to define their precise cause and to decide which model relates more closely to the human situation.

Response of the periodontium to forces exceeding physiological tolerance, stress and the healthy state, or stress with gingivitis

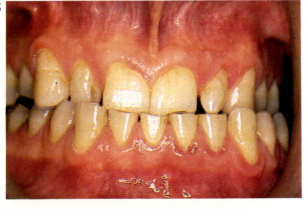

328

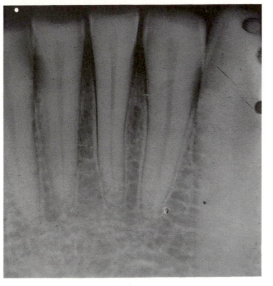

329

328 and 329   Incisor teeth with attrition caused by excessive forces as a result of loss of molar teeth, and radiograph of same teeth showing normal bone height but widening of ligament space and increase in size of the bone trabeculations. The clinical example illustrates the result of research work. Experiments on animals using jiggling forces have shown that such stress neither influenced the degree or extent of gingival inflammation, nor caused apical migration of the junctional epithelium.[1,2] In response to jiggling forces, there was a **traumatic phase** of *developing hypermobility* during which the support structures of teeth subjected to jiggling forces showed an *increasing vascularity*, and a *widening of the periodontal ligament* associated with osteoclastic bone resorption of the inner walls of the socket.[1,2]

After 3-6 months a **post-traumatic phase** was described in which there was no further bone resorption, the osteoclasts being no longer evident. *The support structures of the teeth had adapted to the excessive loads.* Although the teeth were more mobile than before the force was applied, the mobility was not increasing; the widened periodontal ligament remained but did not show further change. This adaptation of the periodontal tissue could be considered as a stable state.

Stress with periodontitis

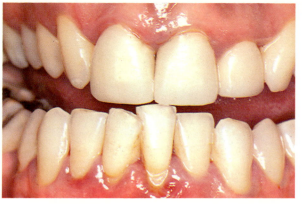

330 and 331 Incisor tooth with periodontitis subjected to heavy load in protrusion, and radiograph of the incisor tooth with combined periodontitis and occlusal trauma. This patient has a lower incisor tooth with periodontitis, subjected to occlusal stress. The effect of jiggling forces on teeth with experimentally-induced periodontitis has been investigated in monkeys,[3] and in dogs.[2] Both studies reported that there was increased mobility when trauma from occlusion was superimposed on periodontitis.

In monkeys, it was found that *combined periodontitis and jiggling forces resulted in a greater reduction in interproximal bone density than periodontitis alone. These changes included a greater loss of bone height, increase in periodontal ligament width and enlargement of trabecular spaces.* Occlusal trauma did not cause greater loss of attachment when superimposed on the periodontitis model in the monkey.

In dogs, a similar study into combined periodontitis with trauma showed additional features; there was greater proliferation of the pocket epithelium. Angular osseous defects in bone were noted on the traumatised teeth, as well as the previous changes described in the alveolar bone for the monkey.

Although these studies were carried out in animals, it may be inferred from them that bone loss in human periodontitis is exacerbated by occlusal trauma, with resultant increase in mobility. The influence of trauma from occlusion with periodontitis on the apical migration of pocket epithelium is controversial; the difference between the results of the studies just quoted may be caused by variation in the forces applied, the species of animal and the type of experimental periodontal bone destruction.

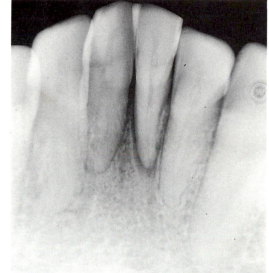

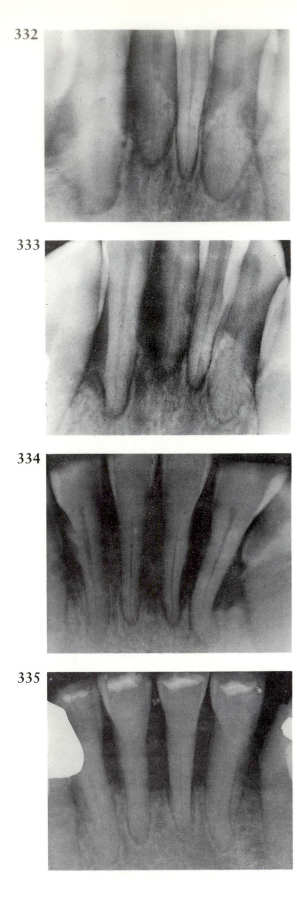

332

333

334

335

Treatment by reduction in occlusal stress only

332 and 333 Radiograph of lower incisor teeth with advanced bone loss, increased width of periodontal ligament and severe mobility, and the same teeth 2 years later after occlusal adjustment and splinting with acid etch composite. The level of plaque control was poor and resolution of inflammation was not achieved. There has been continuing loss of bone.

A review article[4] summarised previous animal studies on occlusion, with emphasis on the priorities for treatment of trauma from occlusion. It was found that removing the traumatogenic forces without treatment of an accompanying periodontitis had no beneficial effect on the periodontal bone. The interproximal bone density continued to deteriorate and the mobility continued to increase.

Treatment by control of bacterial irritants as a priority

334 and 335 Radiograph of incisor teeth with advanced bone loss, increased width of periodontal ligament and severe mobility, and the same teeth 20 years after a complete course of periodontal treatment, comprising plaque control and scaling, with subsequent maintenance. A temporary incisal edge splint was cemented for the first 6 months of therapy.

Following the establishment of combined periodontitis with occlusal trauma, there was an investigation into the combined effects of removing plaque on a regular basis and discontinuing the jiggling forces.[4] It was found that new bone was formed on the socket walls of the previously widened periodontal ligament, and in the narrow spaces of the interproximal bone. There was, however, no repair of bone height. This finding is illustrated clinically in the present radiographic series; there has been marked improvement in bone density and narrowing of the periodontal ligament over the 20-year period. The improvement can be attributed primarily to the patient's excellent plaque control.

In a report[4] on the treatment of combined periodontitis and occlusal trauma by plaque control without occlusal adjustment, it was shown that the degree of bone regeneration was slightly less good than when both forms of treatment were used.

The role of splinting

In a summary[5] of the rationale for splinting teeth, it was shown that the application of jiggling forces causing increased tooth mobility, superimposed on reduced but healthy periodontal tissues, was without effect on the level of connective tissue attachment. It was deduced that, on the grounds of periodontal health, there was no reason to splint mobile teeth after periodontal treatment. Mobility was regarded as an adaptation to excess force. The control of marginal inflammation *per se* would maintain connective tissue attachment levels. The grounds for splinting were limited to:

1 Forces exceeding the adaptive capacity of the periodontium, so that if allowed to continue, further reduction in bone density would result in avulsion of the tooth. Recognition of this problem was based on finding a continually increasing mobility, with no evidence of stability being reached to indicate a state of adaptation.[6]

2 A degree of mobility after adaptation which was not compatible with function, the patient finding that the tooth was too loose to use.[5]

3 The above criteria should be considered when selecting the abutment teeth for dental prostheses and when designing appliances. If, as a result of increased loading by the prostheses, the future abutment teeth are likely to be affected by progressively increasing mobility or by mobility interfering with function, then splinting or a modification of the occlusion should be carried out. This is especially true in the case of teeth that have been previously affected by periodontitis.[6]

4 In the management of patients with advanced periodontitis, tooth movement by orthodontic means may be indicated to improve appearance or function. Provided marginal inflammation is controlled, the local trauma exerted by the orthodontic treatment can be tolerated, even where there has been a severe loss of support.[5] The possible need for permanent retention should always be taken into account before starting treatment.[7]

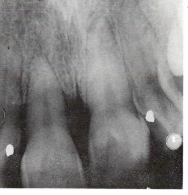

336

336 Localised bone loss on the right central incisor. The right central incisor which was previously affected by localised periodontitis has been treated by preventive methods and by localised periodontal surgery. The patient feels that the tooth is not firm enough for use in normal function. The radiograph shows that only the apical one-third of the root is invested in bone.

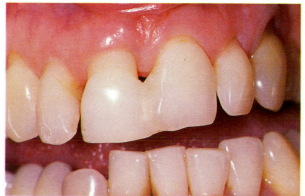

337

337 Clinical appearance of the region. The two central incisor teeth, after acid etching, have been splinted temporarily with composite resin. The patient reports that they are now functionally more satisfactory but, during a thorough discussion on aesthetics, reveals that she is concerned about the degree of over-eruption and the contour of the cervical regions, especially between the right central and lateral incisor teeth.

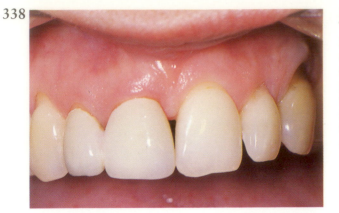

338 **The appearance after fitting splinted crowns.** The patient finds that the splinting of the two right incisor teeth by joined, porcelain bonded to gold crowns has restored her confidence in the function of these teeth. The extra reduction in height of the preparation on the right central incisor has enabled the restoration to be made level with the neighbouring teeth. The cervical contour has been increased to improve aesthetics without adversely encroaching on the embrasure space.

USE OF SPLINTING IN THE COMPLEX TREATMENT PLAN

339 **Chronic periodontitis in the maxillary arch—radiograph.** When the treatment plan for a patient necessitates a multi-disciplined approach, the correct sequence of the various components is crucial to the success of the whole (see Appendix 5). This patient has chronic periodontitis with approximately 2 to 3 mm of interproximal bone destruction.

340 **Chronic periodontitis—clinical appearance.** The maxillary right lateral incisor has begun to migrate labially. This appears to be caused by forces exerted by the tongue and lower lip. The initial phase of therapy has included oral hygiene instruction, and scaling and polishing of the teeth. The patient has achieved good plaque control, but there are residual pockets.

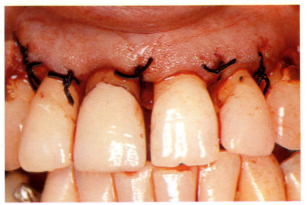

341 **Sutured flap after surgery.** The right lateral incisor has been orthodontically retracted. Periodontal surgery has been carried out subsequently to correct residual pocketing, the labial flap having been apically repositioned to eliminate the pockets.

342 The maxillary restoration using splinted units. The right second premolar and the left first premolar teeth had reduced support as a result of previous periodontal disease. It was considered that the use of these teeth as abutments might exert forces beyond the adaptive capacity of the periodontium. As part of the reconstruction, these abutments were splinted to the neighbouring teeth, thereby redistributing the torque caused by the free-end saddles to the joined teeth, instead of to the relatively poorly supported single units.

   The right lateral incisor, which had been moved orthodontically, is now retained in position by a permanent splint.

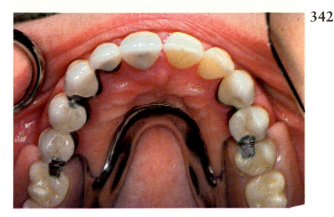

342

The influence of malocclusion and malalignment

343 Periodontal disease involving malaligned teeth. Some studies have reported an increase in periodontal disease associated with malaligned teeth; it was deduced that this association resulted from greater difficulty in removing plaque deposits where tooth alignment was irregular.[8,9] Oral hygiene standards may be considered[10] under three categories: good, moderate and poor. In this patient, who exhibits moderately effective oral hygiene, the gingival condition is less good in the upper right lateral incisor region than elsewhere. As a result of the moderately effective plaque control, the influence of the malaligned teeth on the gingival condition is apparent.

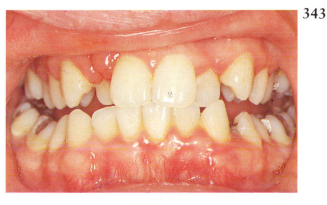

343

344 Malaligned teeth after periodontal treatment. It was observed[10] that patients who had achieved very good standards of oral hygiene were able to remove deposits even from the surfaces of poorly aligned teeth; hence, the gingival condition was uniformly healthy. The patient shown in **343** subsequently completed a course of periodontal treatment. As a result of excellent oral hygiene, gingival health is now being maintained. Special plaque control equipment may be recommended to patients with imbricated teeth, for example, the use of a single-tufted brush (see **148**).

   It was found[10] that where oral hygiene standards were poor, there was no difference in gingival condition between regions with regular or irregular tooth position, as plaque deposits collected indiscriminately on almost all surfaces.

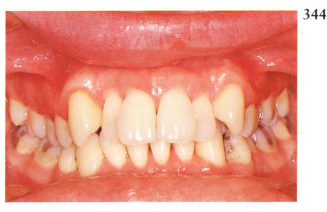

344

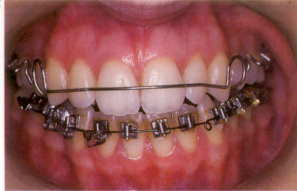

345 **Periodontal implications of orthodontic treatment.** From the above discussion, it is clear that minor tooth malalignment does not pose a major threat to periodontal health provided that the patient responds to specific instruction. Where aesthetic considerations necessitate orthodontic therapy, plaque control is of particular importance during the active phase of treatment as even modern fixed appliances using etched brackets tend to result in increased plaque retention. Previous studies on patients using multiband appliances have shown a transient increase in gingivitis and a greater mean loss of attachment of 0.3 mm during the treatment phase.[11,12,13] It is likely that these disadvantages will be reduced by modern techniques, using brackets which are less plaque-retentive and by careful oral hygiene instruction.[14]

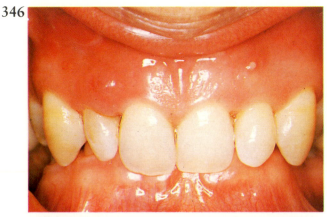

346 **Direct trauma to the palatal gingiva.** The influence of arch relationship on periodontal disease, according to some studies, is not significant.[15] There are clinical situations, however, where increased vertical overbite can cause periodontal damage.[16] On this patient, palatal abscess formation has resulted from direct trauma to the palatal gingiva by the lower incisor teeth, and sinuses are discharging through the buccal alveolar bone in the right and left lateral incisor regions.

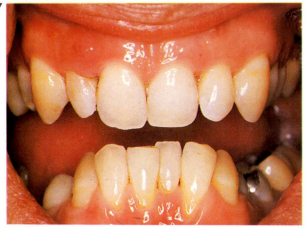

347 **Direct trauma to the mandibular labial gingiva.** Tissue damage to the lower labial gingiva, also, is sometimes found in patients with Angle Class II division ii malocclusion. The changes caused by direct trauma are enhanced by the presence of plaque. A priority when treating these problems is the establishment of good oral hygiene, as subsequent resolution produces soft tissue shrinkage which may reduce the pressure of the tissue contact and, also, the healthy gingiva are more resistant to trauma. For more complex methods of treatment see **311** and **312**.

Treatment of migrating teeth

348 Migrating incisor teeth—periodontitis The patient is concerned about the space between her central incisor teeth which has been increasing for the past 2 years. The first priority in her treatment is the achievement of a plaque control programme.

The migration of periodontally involved teeth is usually caused by several factors. The degree of periodontal destruction is of major significance as the maintenance of the interproximal contacts is jeopardised by any decrease in the quantity or quality of the periodontal support structures, for example, the transeptal gingival fibres or the principal fibres of the periodontal ligament.

349 Adverse lower lip relationship. At rest, the patient's lower lip lies behind the upper incisor teeth. This soft tissue relationship results in an anterior component of force being applied near the tip of the teeth, which is inadequately compensated by the posterior force exerted by the upper lip further apically on the crowns of the teeth.

The patient is concerned by the proclination and spacing of her front teeth; one of her priorities in seeking treatment is aesthetic improvement.

350 Loss of posterior maxillary teeth—anterior slide. On examining the occlusion, it was found that the patient had had several posterior, maxillary teeth extracted on the right-hand side. The remaining teeth had drifted. Examination of the articulation from the retruded contact to the intercuspal position revealed a slide, with a combination of a right lateral and an anterior component.

The central incisor teeth were in contact in the retruded position; mandibular movement from this position into the intercuspal position transmitted, via the lower incisor teeth, an anteriorly directed force to the upper incisors. This type of slide is a common contributory factor in the migration of teeth.[17]

351 Premature contact in retruded position causing anterior slide. A premature contact in the retruded position has been marked with articulating paper. It is found, where there is a slide from retruded contact to the intercuspal position, that the inter-arch tooth contacts causing this anterior movement are on the mesial inclinations of the upper cusps and on the distal inclinations of the lower cusps. This has been termed the 'MUDL' rule.[18]

Small steps are cut into the cuspal inclines at the points of premature contact to provide flat, stable bases for the opposing cusps, and to achieve longer contacts through centric articulation.

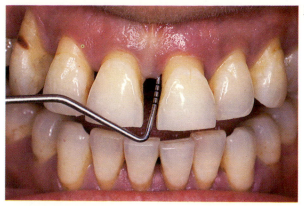

348

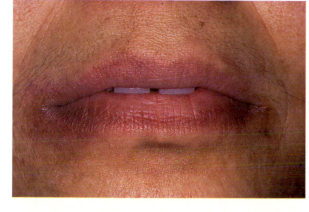

349

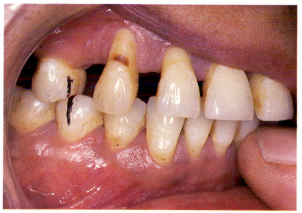

350

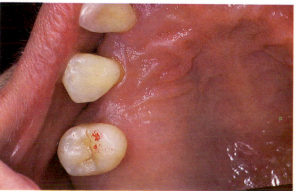

351

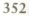

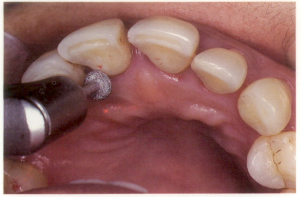

352 Occlusal adjustment—anterior region. The premature contact in the articulation from the retruded position to intercuspation has also been marked. If, as in this case, the teeth have increased mobility it may be necessary to steady the upper incisors, by applying a controlling force labially with the index fingers to achieve a marking of the premature contact. Occlusal adjustment is being carried out using a wheel-shaped diamond stone to cut small step-like ledges on the palatal aspect of the central incisor teeth. This adjustment reduces the interferences on the incisor teeth, thereby eliminating the anterior force on them during the articulation from the retruded position to intercuspation. The contact of the lower incisor teeth with the ledges on the upper teeth prevents over-eruption. It is important not to reduce the height of the lower incisor teeth to eliminate such prematurities, as alteration of contact areas involved in the 'intercuspal stop system' is liable to result in over-eruption.[18]

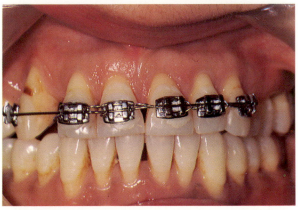

353 Orthodontic treatment. Following the achievement of a plaque control programme, and the equilibration of occlusal forces, orthodontic treatment was used to retract the incisor teeth. The position and root inclination of the canine tooth favoured the enhancement of the existing space between it and the lateral incisor tooth, with the future provision of a pontic rather than the alternative of closing this space. The use of orthodontic forces on treated periodontally involved teeth does not jeopardise the periodontium, provided plaque control is carefully monitored and maintained. Clearly, recurrence of periodontitis with orthodontic treatment in progress would be very damaging as, in effect, it would be equivalent to the phenomenon of trauma with periodontitis.

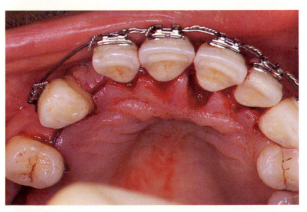

354 Periodontal surgery—palatal aspect. The periodontal condition was checked after the active phase of orthodontic treatment. Residual pockets were found, which bled on probing. Periodontal surgery was carried out on the palatal aspect, an inverse bevel incision with enhanced scalloping being used. The saddle areas were modified by thinning the tissue.

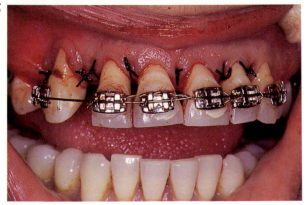

355 Periodontal surgery—labial aspect after suturing. The periodontal surgery on the labial aspect was conservative, an inverse bevel intrasulcular incision being used on the marginal aspects. For the interproximal papillae, an inverse bevel incision was used to thin the hyperplastic corium while retaining as much of the keratinised gingiva on the labial aspect as possible. The flap has been replaced at the original level and sutured.

356 Acid-etched bridge and splint—palatal. The upper anterior segment has been treated with a combined splint and bridge to act as a permanent retainer after the orthodontic treatment and to provide a pontic to fill the space between the right canine and lateral incisor teeth. The prosthesis was retained with composite resin on acid-etched abutment teeth. The palatal aspect of the prosthesis was adjusted to prevent occlusal interferences. The resultant step-like ledges can be seen.

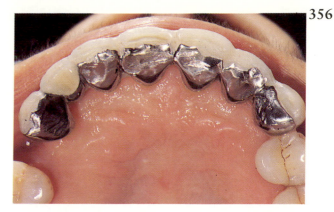

357 Acid-etched bridge and splint—labial. The incisor teeth have been retracted sufficiently by the orthodontic treatment so that, when relaxed, the lower lip rests on the labial aspect of these teeth. The spaces between the teeth have been closed and the patient is pleased with the appearance. She will have a bridge made for the upper right posterior segment now and is on a continuing maintenance programme for the preventive aspects of treatment.

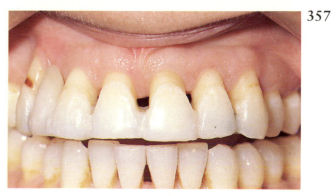

17 PERIODONTICS AND RESTORATIVE DENTISTRY

The junction between even an ideal restoration and a tooth will appear rough at the microscopic level and this surface roughness will result in plaque being retained, in spite of the oral hygiene measures practised by the patient. The subgingival placement of cavity margins causes enhanced inflammation and periodontitis, as a result of the associated increase in irritants retained in contact with the soft tissue. Poor quality margins and, especially, overhangs exacerbate this damaging effect.[1,2]

Preventive periodontal treatment is a valuable preliminary to restorative treatment as gingival hyperplasia can be reduced, and the associated bleeding and gingival exudate can be eliminated, reducing the possible contamination of restorative materials. More complex measures including periodontal surgery or, less commonly, orthodontic extrusion may be indicated also, to enable restorations to be placed in the correct relationship to healthy periodontal tissue.[3,4]

Endodontic assessment is often necessary to determine the nature of a particular lesion. The diagnosis will influence the type of treatment to be used. Some of the more elaborate periodontal treatment techniques require prior elective endodontic therapy, for example, in the case of root resection on molar teeth (**286** to **297**).

Where there is severe loss of periodontal attachment, as part of the overall periodontal treatment, restorations on neighbouring teeth may be splinted together. Fixed or removable prosthetic appliances may be designed with a view to stabilising teeth.[5] The indications for splinting are defined and some examples are shown (see **336** to **342**).

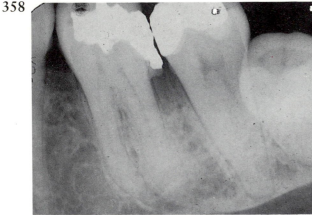

358

The correction of plaque retentive margins and the treatment of associated periodontal problems

NON-SURGICAL TREATMENT

358 Amalgam restoration with overhang at margin. The radiograph shows a defective amalgam restoration with excess amalgam cervically, resulting in an overhang. Subsequently, when this segment of the arch was being treated by root planing, the overhang was trimmed with a sharpened scaling instrument and smoothed with a diamond point in a reciprocating handpiece.[6,7] The margin of the restoration was checked, using a probe and dental floss to ensure that it was smooth. A plaque control regime was implemented. The third molar tooth was extracted to prevent the possible future loss of distal bone on the second molar tooth.

359 **The same restoration as shown in 358, one year after recontouring.** Twelve months after the smoothing of the restoration and with continuing plaque control there is evidence of increased density in the associated interproximal bone. The socket of the third molar tooth has healed and the distal pocket on the second molar tooth has resolved.

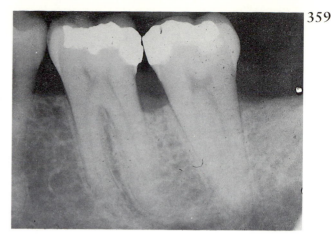

The correction of restorations with defective margins and the setting up of a comprehensive periodontal preventive programme will usually result in the resolution of inflammation, and this may be accompanied by shrinkage of the swollen gingival margins so that they are no longer in contact with the restorations. If necessary, defective restorations can be replaced, but such replacement should be deferred until the periodontal condition has improved. At this stage, the level of the gingival margin will be stabilised, and the new restoration can be placed under the best possible conditions of access and with minimal gingival bleeding or exudate.

Applications of surgical procedures in restorative dentistry

A plan to undertake the provision of new or replacement crowns or bridges should always involve a thorough periodontal assessment. Prior periodontal treatment may be restricted to preventive periodontal procedures but periodontal surgery may be indicated where inflammation and pocketing persist after the initial phase of periodontal treatment. Other indications for surgery include the presence of subgingival caries or restorations, and inadequate access for the restorative work (see also **232** to **241**). It may be found that, as a result of previous loss of tooth tissue, there is an inadequate width of extra-alveolar cementum, so that the necessary zone for the attachment of gingival fibres and junctional epithelium is not available. Osseous surgery is then indicated to achieve a band of at least 2 mm of extra-alveolar cementum, and preferably as much as 4 mm. The restorative dentist may also require increased clinical crown height to assist retention.

360 **Inadequate bridges—gingival inflammation.** Some years ago, the patient had bridges constructed to replace the congenitally absent lateral incisor teeth. The margins of these bridges were unsatisfactory and there is now gingival hyperplasia with about 5 mm of pocketing and bleeding on probing. The patient has undertaken a course of plaque control for several months but there has been minimal improvement of the periodontal condition.

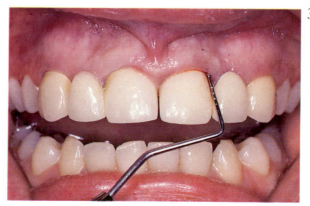

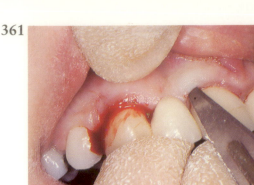

361 Conservative inverse bevel incision. The condition is being treated by periodontal surgery to re-establish the correct dento-gingival relationships. A conservative inverse bevel incision is being outlined at the crest of the gingiva. The aim is to retain the maximum width of gingival tissue as the patient is anxious to keep postsurgical recession to a minimum.

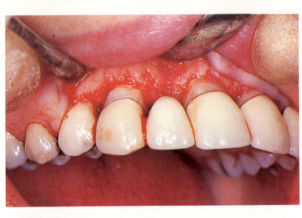

362 Surgical treatment—bone contour. Curettage and root planing have been completed. The width of supra-alveolar cementum was assessed; there was the necessary 2-3 mm width to allow for both the insertion of new gingival fibres and the formation of a new junctional epithelial attachment. Where there is not an adequate width of cementum present, periodontal bone at the crest of the alveolus has to be removed with chisels (see **373**).

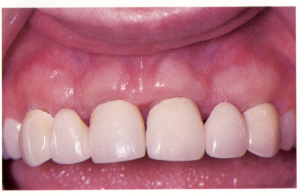

363 Healing 12 weeks after surgery. Twelve weeks after surgery, new bridges are being assessed at the try-in stage. There is a 2 mm sulcus depth and the new crowns have been prepared so that the margins are level with the gingiva. Ideally, definitive preparations for crowns should not be made until about 20 weeks after periodontal surgery.[8] It has been found that there is a coronal movement of the gingival crest for the first 6 weeks after surgery, followed by gradual apical movement which stabilised at 20 weeks.

Prosthetic dentistry

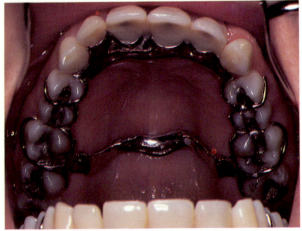

364 Partial dental prosthesis with minimal tissue coverage. The wearing of a dental prosthesis inevitably increases plaque retention. This effect can be minimised by giving the patient oral hygiene instruction, with particular emphasis on cleaning the area covered by the prosthesis.[9,10,11]

A tooth-borne design of prosthesis, as shown, with minimal gingival cover is well tolerated by the periodontal tissues.

365 Tissue-borne acrylic partial prosthesis. This tissue-borne acrylic denture has many design faults; there are no clasps or occlusal rests and there is excessive coverage of the gingival margins. The prosthesis has been worn for 6 years without being relined.

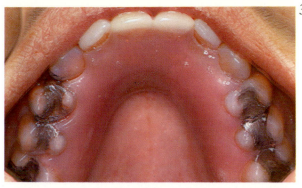

366 Soft tissue response to prolonged retention of irritants. Enhanced plaque retention at the gingival margins has resulted in gingival hyperplasia and periodontitis. Overgrowth of *Candida albicans* micro-organisms may also be a problem. Gingival proliferation will be enhanced if there is any space between the appliance and the soft tissues.[12] It is important to achieve a healthy periodontium before making a new prosthesis.

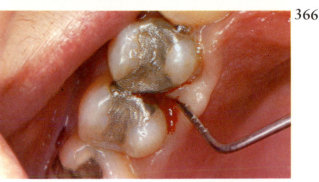

366

367 Radiograph of the involved teeth. There has been 1-2 mm of bone loss in the upper right molar region as a result of the prolonged inflammation. There are no obvious bone defects on the radiograph.

The initial plaque control phase of treatment resulted in some reduction of inflammation. The patient was encouraged to take out the denture at night. It was considered that periodontal surgery was needed to remove the fibrous, hyperplastic gingiva.

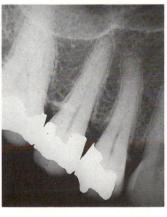

367

368 Palatal aspect after periodontal surgery At this stage, periodontal surgery has been carried out. The pockets have been eliminated and there is a satisfactory contour. A new prosthesis is to be constructed. This will be a cobalt chrome partial denture and will have minimal soft tissue coverage (see **364**).

A regular recall system is necessary to ensure adequate maintenance of the periodontal condition of patients who wear dentures.[13]

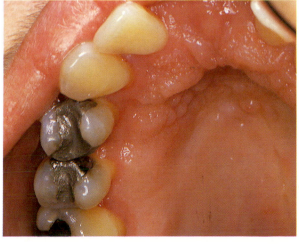

368

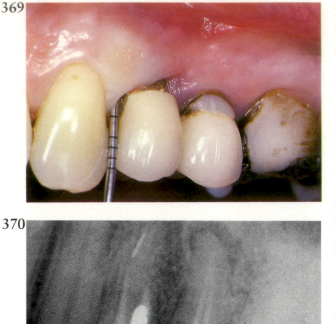

More complex periodontal treatment in relation to restorative dentistry

SURGICAL ENDODONTICS COMBINED WITH PERIODONTAL SURGERY

369   Periodontal pocketing on teeth that are to be recrowned. The patient has had these crowns for about 6 years. His plaque control has been generally only fair, and the poor crown margins accentuated the local retention of plaque with resultant periodontitis. He has completed a plaque control programme, with special emphasis on interproximal cleaning. There are residual 5 mm pockets.

370   Radiograph of the premolar teeth. This shows that the endodontic treatment is inadequate and there are periapical radiolucencies around the apices of both premolar teeth. It is planned to perform surgical-endodontic treatment as a joint procedure with the periodontal surgery.

371   Inverse bevel incision. This is being used to gain access to the surgical site on the labial aspect and, similarly, on the palatal aspect. When making the incisions, the objectives are to thin the interproximal papillae and to achieve a tapered scalloped outline.

372   After curettage has been completed. A relieving incision was used to enable localised apical repositioning of the gingiva to be achieved. It will also enhance access, which is especially advantageous in this case, where surgical-endodontic treatment is to be performed.

373 Access for apical surgery. Further elevation of the flap was carried out. It was found that there were localised areas where the width of supra-alveolar cementum was less than the 2-4 mm considered necessary for insertion of new gingival fibres, and for the formation of a new junctional epithelial attachment. At the relevant sites, a chisel was used to reduce the crestal bone height. It was necessary to be very conservative in bone removal where a furcation might be involved, for example, in the interproximal region of the first premolar tooth. Adequate reflection of the flap has been achieved for the endodontic procedures. Both the premolar teeth have been treated by apicectomy and retrograde root treatment.

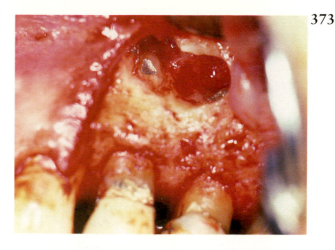

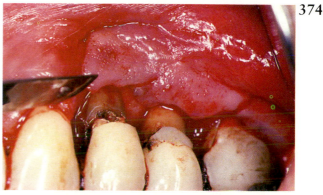

374 Apical repositioning of the flap. The repositioning of the flap is now being judged. It is planned to reposition the flap apically by about 2 mm, so that the soft tissues will be clear of the margins of the crowns and the bone margins will be just covered by the flap. A small step at the relieving incision would result from this repositioning; a triangle of marginal tissue is being removed to correct this potential anomaly before suturing.

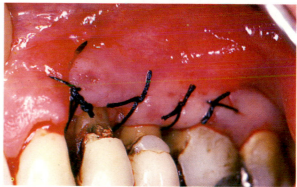

375 The flap has been sutured. The suturing technique at the relieving incision is important. The needle was initially passed through the flap, close to the tip of the papilla. The needle was then taken through the fixed labial gingiva at a more apical level, near the muco-gingival junction. The resultant inclination of the suture across the line of incision resulted in the flap being pulled apically when the suture was tightened. Interrupted sutures were then placed. An additional, more apical suture is to be placed to complete the closure at the relieving incision.

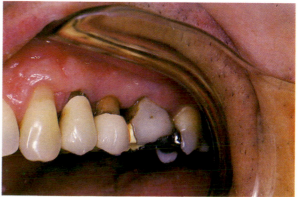

376 Postoperative healing. The gingivae have healed well. The apically repositioned flap has provided very good access for subsequent restorative treatment. The pockets have been eliminated. The periodontal treatment is now centred on preventive maintenance. The patient will need advice about the management of plaque control around the new crowns, when these have been completed.

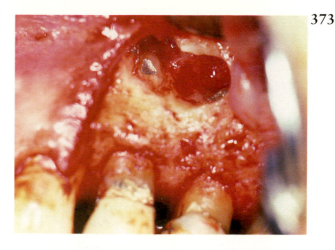

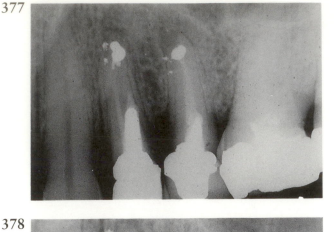

377 Postoperative radiograph. A postoperative radiograph was taken to confirm the adequacy of the retrograde root treatments. It will be used, also, for follow-up to enable subsequent periapical bone regeneration to be assessed.

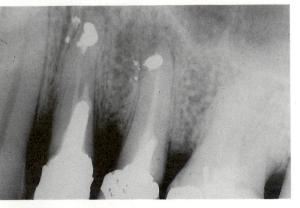

378 Three-month follow-up. The 3-month follow-up radiograph shows a reduction in the size of the periapical radiolucency. It is concluded that the endodontic surgery has been successful.

Indication for bridge on treated teeth that have lost periodontal support

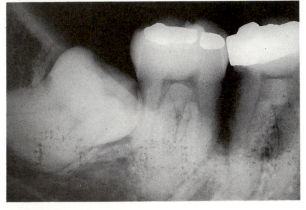

379 Radiograph before treatment—severe bone loss. Before treatment, the patient had severe alveolar bone loss on all the teeth in the mandibular right posterior segment. There was bifurcation involvement on the first molar tooth. The third molar tooth was impacted and needed to be extracted.

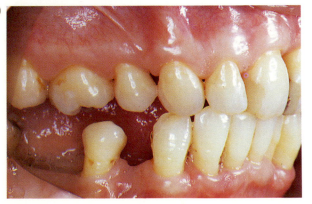

380 Clinical condition after periodontal treatment and extractions. The severely involved teeth have been extracted and the periodontal treatment, including periodontal surgery, has been completed. The teeth are now being assessed with a view to constructing a bridge. It has been found that even teeth with severely reduced bone support can be used as abutments, provided they receive prior periodontal treatment and very good plaque control is maintained.[14,15]

381 The completed bridge. The bridge was designed with supra-gingival margins. Although there was in excess of Grade I mobility, the condition was stable with no sign of increase in mobility at subsequent visits. The plaque control is under regular maintenance.

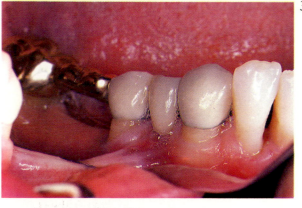

381

382 Post-treatment radiograph at 18 months. The condition of the periodontal bone appears to be satisfactory. The crestal bone seems dense and the height stable relative to the previous radiographs.

382

ORTHODONTIC EXTRUSION

383 Subgingival fracture. This canine tooth of a 22-year-old female patient has recently fractured, about 3 mm of the root being involved by the fracture line on the palatal aspect. The objective is to achieve an extrusion of the tooth and convert the subgingival margins to supragingival.[4]

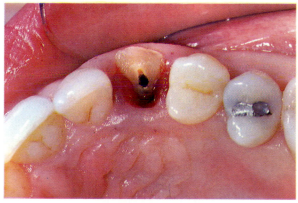

383

384 Radiograph of the tooth. The tooth had excellent periodontal support and an adequate root length. A previously placed sectional root treatment appeared clinically to be satisfactory.

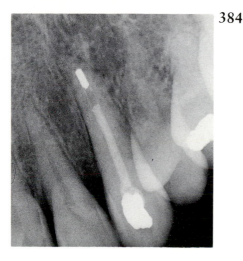

384

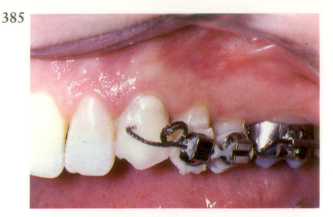

385   Orthodontic appliance. A temporary crown was placed, using a dentine screw in the root canal; a severely compromised palatal marginal fit was accepted for the present. A fixed orthodontic appliance was then used to induce orthodontic extrusion.

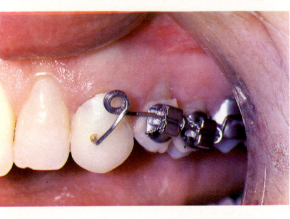

386   After orthodontic extrusion. The degree of orthodontic extrusion can be gauged by the change in angle of the arm of the appliance. The temporary crown has been ground down to reduce the height as extrusion proceeded. It was necessary to hold the tooth in retention for several months to prevent relapse. It is interesting to note that, as the tooth was orthodontically extruded, the gingival margin moved with the tooth.[16]

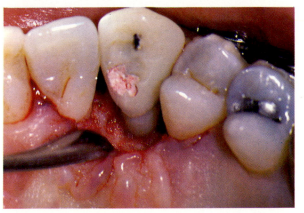

387   Assessing bone contours. At the time of surgery it was found that, as a result of the orthodontic extrusion, the bone level on all aspects of the canine tooth was at a more coronal level relative to the neighbouring teeth.[16] On the palatal aspect, after the extrusion phase the fracture line was still located subgingivally. At this stage, minor osseous surgery was carried out to achieve a 2-4 mm width of cementum for the attachment of both gingival fibres and junctional epithelium.

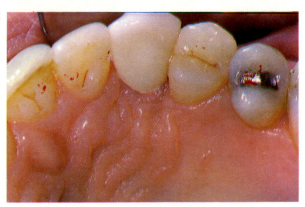

388   Palatal aspect after new crown. A post crown has been constructed with margins level with the gingival crest palatally. The tissue contour relative to the neighbouring teeth is acceptable.

389 Labial aspect after new crown. The appearance of the crown is satisfactory. In this case, if orthodontic extrusion had not been used, the degree of surgical correction necessary to expose the margins would have resulted in severe post-operative recession, involving both the palatal gingiva and, of greater consequence aesthetically, the papillae.

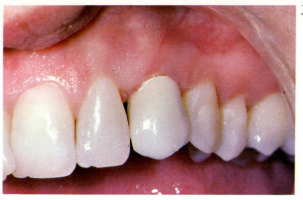

Appendix 1
CLASSIFICATION OF PERIODONTAL DISEASES

(see also factors which alter host response—Appendix 2)

Periodontal diseases	Associated micro-organisms
1) Gingivitis	
Acute necrotising ulcerative gingivitis	Treponema, *Bacteroides intermedius*, Fusobacteria
Gingival abscess	(Response to impacted foreign object)
Chronic gingivitis	Species of: Streptococci, Fusobacteria, Actinomyces, Treponema, Bacteroides
2) Periodontitis	
Periodontal abscess	Gram-negative anaerobic organisms
Chronic adult periodontitis	*Wolinella recta, Bacteroides intermedius, B. gingivalis, B. forsythus, Fusobacterium nucleatum*
Prepubertal periodontitis	Gram-negative cocci and rods
Juvenile periodontitis	*Actinobacillus actinomycetemcomitans, Capnocytophaga gingivalis*
Rapidly progressive periodontitis	*Bacteroides gingivalis, Actinobacillus actinomycetemcomitans*
Refractory periodontitis	*Actinobacillus actinomycetemcomitans, Bacteroides gingivalis*

Appendix 2
AETIOLOGY AND PATHOGENESIS OF PERIODONTAL DISEASES

Plaque formation
Salivary components
Micro-organisms
Substrate (from food)

Local protective factors
Saliva ⟨ Diluting action
Antibacterial action
Dento-gingival form
Junctional epithelial attachment
Epithelial cell turnover
Gingival fluid

Inflammatory response
Vascular changes
Cellular exudate

Humoral immune response
(B-lymphocytes, plasma cells)
Antibodies to bacteria,
proteins other antigens
Antibody + antigen →
complex
Complement cascade
Release of active products:
anaphlatoxin, chemotactic
agents, opsonins, lytic agents
to bacteria

Cellular immune response
(T-, B-lymphocytes, lymphokines)
Inhibit macrophage migration
Inhibit migration of mononuclear cells
Cause lysis of sensitised cells
Activate osteoclasts

Polymorphonuclear leukocytes

Macrophages
Phagocytosis, release of lysosomal
enzymes and prostaglandins

**Metabolites from plaque
micro-organisms**
Endotoxins, lipoteichoic acid
Enzymes
Antigens
Other chemicals: ammonia,
hydrogen sulphide, toxic
amines

**Factors which alter the host
response**
Blood dyscrasias:
Leukaemia
Agranulocytosis
Cyclic neutropenia

Drugs
Hydantoin
Nifedipine
Cyclosporin
Other immunosuppressive drugs
Contraceptive hormones

Hormonal changes
Puberty
Pregnancy
Menopause
Diabetes

Appendix 3
PERIODONTAL INDICES

Epidemiological studies have been carried out on a variety of population groups to assess the level of periodontal diseases and link them to various causative factors. Clinical epidemiology, also, has been used to assess the effectiveness of a variety of treatment procedures.

Current periodontal research has been made possible only by the development of a variety of indices, consisting of a series of definitions designed to record the status of the periodontal tissues and aetiological agents. These may be used to give an indication of the types of treatment needed. The index measurements may be applied in several ways:

(a) Multiple surfaces on each tooth—Gingival Index,[1] Plaque Index,[2] which are recorded on 4 surfaces of each tooth.
(b) On every tooth—Periodontal Index.[3]
(c) On selected teeth—Periodontal Disease Index,[4] which records disease on 6 representative teeth.
(d) On segments—Community Periodontal Index of treatment needs,[5] where the most severely involved tooth is measured in each sextant.

1 Oral hygiene indices

The oral hygiene indices are generally based on 2 concepts: the proportion of the crown of the tooth covered with plaque (a), or the quantity of plaque in proximity to gingival margins (b). The latter may seem more relevant in studies of periodontal diseases.

(a) Oral Hygiene Index (Greene and Vermillion 1960)[6]
0 No debris or stain
1 Soft debris covering not more than one-third of the tooth surface
2 Soft debris covering more than one-third, but not more than two-thirds of tooth surface
3 Soft debris covering over two-thirds of tooth surface.

(b) Plaque Index (Silness and Loe 1964)[2]
0 No plaque
1 Film of plaque, visible only by removal on probe or by disclosing
2 Moderate accumulation of deposits within the pockets or on the margins which can be seen with the naked eye
3 Heavy accumulation of soft material filling the niche between gingival margin and tooth surface. Interdental region is filled with debris.

2 Plaque retention indices

Retention Index (Loe 1967)[7]
0 No caries, calculus or imperfect margin of restorations in a gingival location
1 Supragingival calculus, cavity or imperfect margin
2 Subgingival calculus, cavity or imperfect margin
3 Large cavity abundance of calculus or grossly imperfect margin.

3 Gingival indices

Measurements of gingivitis are based on 3 principles:
(a) Whether inflammation is at local points only on the gingival circumference, or whether it circumscribes the tooth completely
(b) Assessment of a combination of colour change, contour change and bleeding on probing at defined sites
(c) Assessment of bleeding on probing by various criteria.

The Gingival Index (Loe and Silness 1963)[1]
0 Normal gingiva
1 Mild inflammation, slight change in colour, slight oedema, no bleeding on probing
2 Moderate inflammation, redness, oedema and glazing; bleeding on probing
3 Severe inflammation, marked redness and oedema, ulceration; tendency to spontaneous haemorrhage.

Papillary Bleeding Index (Muhlemann 1977)[8]
PBI Index based on bleeding following gentle probing of the interdental papilla
0 No bleeding
1 Only 1 bleeding point present
2 Several isolated bleeding points or a small area of blood
3 Interdental triangle filled with blood
4 Profuse bleeding spreading towards the marginal gingiva.

4 Combined indices of gingivitis and periodontitis

This group of indices has been designed to measure both gingivitis and periodontitis with the most emphasis on the destructive phases of disease.

Recently there has been a change towards separating the measurement of periodontitis, this being determined by measurement of loss of attachment from the enamel-cement junction or bone loss on radiographs.

The Periodontal Index (Russell 1956)[3]

0 There is neither overt inflammation in the investing tissue nor loss of function due to destruction of supporting tissue. Radiographic appearance is normal.
1 Mild gingivitis. There is an overt area of inflammation in the free gingiva but this area does not circumscribe the tooth.
2 Gingivitis. Inflammation completely circumscribes the tooth but there is no apparent break in the epithelial attachment.
4 (Not used in field studies). There is an early notch-like resorption of the alveolar crest.
6 Gingivitis with pocket formation. The epithelial attachment has been broken and there is a pocket (not merely a deepened gingival crevice caused by swelling in the free gingiva). There is no interference with normal masticatory function, the tooth is firm in its socket and has not drifted. Radiographically, there is bone loss involving the entire alveolar crest up to half of the length of the tooth root (distance from apex to enamel-cement junction).
8 Advanced destruction with loss of masticatory function. The tooth may be loose, may have drifted, may sound dull on percussion with a metallic instrument, may be depressible in its socket. Radiographically, there is advanced bone loss involving more than one-half of the length of the tooth root, or a definite widening of the periodontal membrane. There may be root resorption or rarefaction at the apex.
RULE: When in doubt, assign the lesser score.

Peridontal Disease Index (Ramfjord 1959)[4]

This index is recorded by measurements taken on the following teeth 6 /1 4 and 4 1/ 6. The use of representative teeth reduces the number of measurements.
0 Health
1 Mild to moderate inflammatory change not extending all around tooth
2 Mild to moderate inflammatory change extending all around tooth
3 Severe gingivitis, characterised by marked redness, tendency to bleed, ulceration
4 3 mm apical extension of crevice from enamel-cement junction
5 3-6 mm extension
6 Over 6 mm extension.

5 Indices of treatment needs

The objective of these indices is strictly related to treatment aspects. The limitations must be borne in mind so that they are not used in place of indices designed to measure levels of disease.

The Community Periodontal Index of Treatment Needs (Ainamo 1988)[5]

In this index the worst score is recorded for each of 6 segments. A special CPITN probe is necessary and treatment required for each segment is based on the score recorded (see **137**).

1 Gingival bleeding but no pocket, no calculus, no overhanging restoration. Patient needs only OH education.
2 Deepest pocket < 3 mm, sub-gingival calculus present or sub-gingival retention site. Patient needs scaling plus OH education.
3 Deepest pocket 4 or 5 mm which can be managed by deep scaling and OH education.
4 One or more tooth in a sextant has a pocket > 6 mm. Patient needs curettage and root planing at either closed or open operation.

6 Clinical measurements

Several different measurements are used clinically, including measurements of aetiological agents, gingivitis, periodontal pocketing, gingival recession and tooth mobility.

Plaque Control Record (O'Leary, Drake and Taylor 1972)[9]

Four surfaces on each tooth recorded for presence or absence of plaque. Total score of surfaces affected is then expressed as a percentage (see **139**).

Bleeding on Probing Record

This is compiled in the same way as the plaque control record and is useful in monitoring a patient's progress.

Index of Tooth Mobility (see **131** and **132**)[10,11]

Mobility is scored 0 to 3
0 No detectable mobility
1 Barely distinguishable mobility
2 Crown moves up to 1 mm in any direction
3 Crown moves over 1 mm in any direction including depression or rotation

Appendix 4
PERIODONTAL ASSESSMENT FORMS

The use of assessment forms as illustrated facilitates both documenting the patient's history and recording the clinical examination. The forms are useful for the assistant when taking notes, and the layout presents the case record under clear headings. The incorporated grids may be used for recording aetiological agents, inflammation, pockets and the mobility of teeth.

For a more complex case the periodontal chart may be used. This chart is of particular benefit if completed before embarking on the more advanced stages of treatment. The residual pockets should be marked on the chart and these can then be related to the anatomy of the soft tissues and the radiographic picture. Charting also enables the distribution of periodontal disease to be related to local plaque-retaining factors. Where periodontal surgery is indicated, the planning of the order of treatment is facilitated by having the distribution of the pockets presented graphically.

Outline charts in this appendix are provided so that copies may be taken for clinical use.

PERIODONTAL ASSESSMENT FORM   REFERENCE NUMBER

NAME   DATE

ADDRESS   DATE OF BIRTH

COMPLAINT

HISTORY OF COMPLAINT

ORAL HISTORY

ORAL HYGIENE METHODS

MEDICAL HISTORY

SOCIAL HISTORY

EXTRA ORAL EXAMINATION

INTRA ORAL EXAMINATION

MUCOSA / FRENAE

GINGIVAE

PLAQUE

CALCULUS—SUPRAGINGIVAL

SUBGINGIVAL

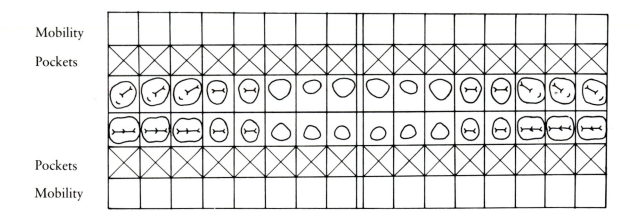

| Mobility | | | | | | | | | | | | | | | | |

Pockets

Pockets

Mobility

OCCLUSION

RADIOGRAPHIC ASSESSMENT

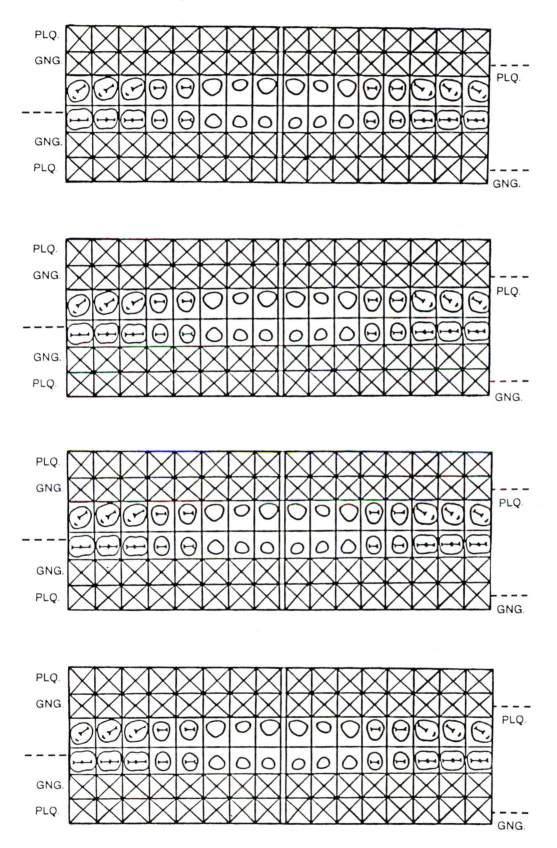

DATE

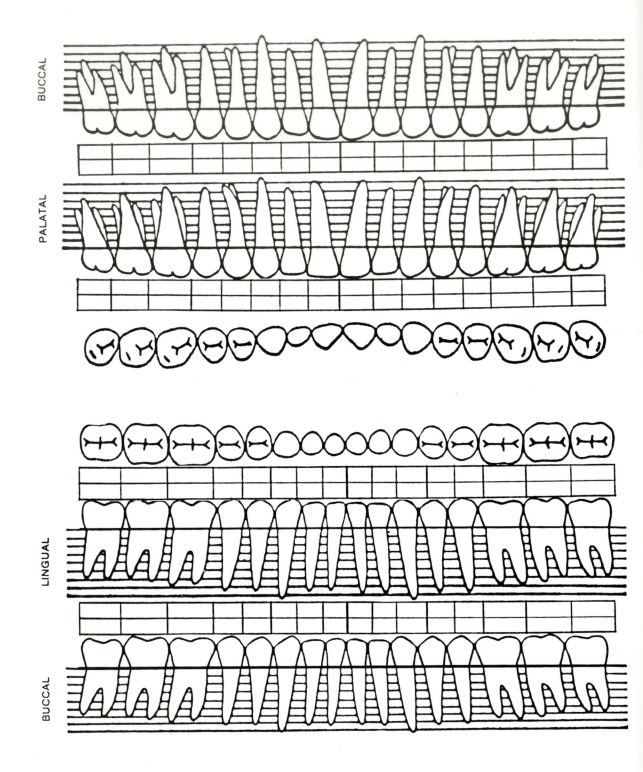

SUMMARY OF DIAGNOSIS AND AETIOLOGY

PROGNOSIS

INITIAL TREATMENT

ADVANCED TREATMENT AND PERIODONTAL SURGERY

Appendix 5
SEQUENCE FOR THE COMPONENTS OF TREATMENT AND MAINTENANCE

History and assessment
Initial therapy:
(a) Oral hygiene instruction
(b) Scaling, polishing and root planning
(c) Smoothing margins of restorations
(d) Replacing unsatisfactory plastic restorations
(e) Occlusal adjustment
(f) Other restorative treatment (endodontics)
(g) Extractions
(h) Transitional crowns
(i) Transitional bridges/prostheses

Full periodontal chart
The initial therapy will have resulted in resolution of inflammation for many patients. Careful selection is necessary to determine suitability for more complex procedures.

Advanced therapy
(a) Orthodontic treatment
(b) Periodontal surgery
(c) Advanced restorative procedures
(d) Prosthetic reconstruction

Order of treatment
The various components of treatment may be transposed where this is indicated but, in general, the procedures in the second group should not be undertaken until those in the first group have been completed.

Periodontal surgery should precede advanced restorative procedures, as the margins of the restorations should be planned in relation to a stabilised gingival level.

Maintenance phase
On completion of therapy, regular maintenance visits are necessary. The frequency of these appointments is determined by the quality of the patient's plaque control over successive visits and by the amount of any inflammation present.

The routine for a maintenance visit comprises:

(a) Recording of plaque and, if relevant, inflammation and pockets.
(b) If areas of defective plaque control are evident, the patient should be asked to demonstrate routine oral hygiene procedures in these areas. The patient can then be guided through the modification in technique necessary to achieve satisfactory results.
(c) All plaque and calculus are removed, special emphasis being placed on removing bacterial deposits from any residual pockets and from the less accessible areas. Periodic meticulous cleaning of plaque from all the tooth surfaces by the clinician has been shown to be of major importance in reinforcing the work by the patient in maintaining periodontal health.
(d) Any symptoms are assessed, and the patient's general dental condition reviewed. Where necessary further treatment is arranged.

Appendix 6
TREATMENT OF CONTAMINATED CEMENTUM

A review[1] describes the various changes detectable in cementum that has been involved by periodontal disease. Plaque and calculus deposits are present on the surface and frequently also in surface resorption lacunae. Other changes include the penetration of toxic substances from plaque into the surface layer of cementum, and hypermineralisation of the surface layer. The appearance of granules and alterations in the organic component have also been reported. Although the precise mechanism has not been defined, several studies have shown that cementum affected by periodontitis is cytotoxic to cells in contact with it.

Various techniques have been described for the removal of this cytotoxic material and to make the surface more compatible for the attachment of host cells. The most commonly used technique is scaling and root planing, to remove plaque and calculus together with the superficial layer of cementum which has been involved by periodontitis.

The application of various substances to the involved root surface following scaling has also been investigated. The aim is to achieve chemical decontamination and to enhance the adhesion of host cells to the treated surface during healing. The materials used have included sodium deoxycholate, Cohn plasma fraction IV, sodium lauryl sulphate with EDTA, sodium hypochlorite, immune serum globulin, fibronectin and citric acid.[2,3,4,5]

Considerable research has centred on the use of citric acid, as this material has not only an anti-bacterial and detoxifying effect but also demineralises dentine or cementum to expose the collagen fibres of the matrix.[6,7,8]

Epithelium may be prevented from migrating apically along denuded root surfaces treated with citric acid by a fibrin network attached to the root surface by an arcade-like structure.[9] The earlier work in animals has met with mixed results when repeated in human research. One study has shown fibrous tissue attaching perpendicularly to either old or newly formed cementum on some of the decalcified root surfaces, but not on the controls.[10] Other studies have shown minimal effect on connective tissue attachment.[11,12]

Current techniques for preparing root surfaces that have been involved by periodontal disease is restricted to thorough mechanical instrumentation and washing with water or saline. The objective is to remove residual plaque and calculus along with the surface layer of cementum which harbours cytotoxic material. This may be done using sharpened curettes, several overlapping strokes being applied to each aspect of the tooth. Extra care is necessary if root morphology is irregular.

Appendix 7
LOCAL ANALGESIA IN PERIODONTAL THERAPY

CHOICE OF ANALGESIC

The analgesic preparation in general use for dental procedures is 2 per cent lignocaine with adrenaline 1 in 80,000. This is available in cartridges which usually contain 2 ml of the solution, although other capacities are available. Injection of solution into a blood vessel can be avoided by using an aspirating syringe.

Alternative analgesic preparations have been developed, for example 3 per cent prilocaine with felypressin 0.03 units per ml. These are of value for the treatment of patients who might react adversely to the lignocaine with adrenaline preparation. For example, an analgesic solution which does not contain adrenaline is preferable for patients with cardiovascular disease, hypertension, hyperthyroidism or who are taking tricyclic antidepressants. The disadvantage of the prilocaine with felypressin preparation is that haemorrhage control is not as good.[1]

INJECTION SITES FOR LOCAL ANALGESIA

It has been shown[2] that local infiltration of analgesic provides better control of haemorrhage during periodontal surgery than the use of nerve block analgesia. To reduce pain, as few injection sites as possible should be used to achieve initial analgesia. On the facial aspect, after the initial penetration of the mucosa, the needle is advanced horizontally through the tissues at the level of the apices of the teeth (see **197**). Analgesic solution is slowly injected ahead of the needle. Three injection sites are usually required for each quadrant on the vestibular aspect. On the palatal and lingual aspects, the analgesic solution is infiltrated at strategic points in relation to the nerve supply of the area.

When initial analgesia has been obtained, and where surgical procedures are to be performed further solution is infiltrated into the papilla and the marginal gingiva associated with each tooth. This reinforces the analgesia and results in further vasoconstriction (see **198**).

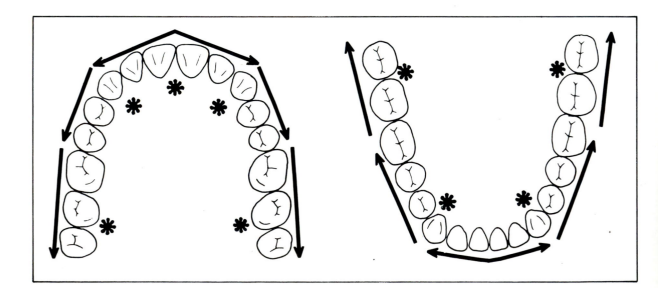

Appendix 8
INDICATIONS FOR SURGERY AND PATIENT MANAGEMENT

The fundamentals of periodontal treatment are the elimination of existing disease and the prevention of its recurrence by suitable postoperative care.

Scaling, rooting planing and polishing, supported by good oral hygiene will result in improvement in inflammation and pocketing and, for many patients, there will be complete resolution of disease.[1,2,3,4,5] In others, despite skilful treatment and diligent home care, there will be residual pockets which bleed on probing.

During initial treatment, assessments should be repeated at intervals to determine co-operation by, and ability of the patient in oral hygiene procedures and to evaluate the response of the periodontal tissues to treatment. It has been shown[6] that the deeper the initial pockets, the less feasible it is to remove all deposits by scaling and root planing with indirect access. It has also been shown[7] that sites which continue to bleed on probing, or show suppuration, are more likely to exhibit further loss of probing attachment in the absence of more complex treatment. Patients with residual pockets displaying these characteristics should be assessed with a view to performing periodontal surgery. This allows direct access to the root surfaces for treatment and also provides the opportunity to eliminate or reduce pockets, and so render previously unreachable tooth surfaces accessible to plaque control measures by the patient. On sites with pre-operative probing depths less than about 4 mm, it has been found that there was a relatively favourable attachment level after treatment by root planing compared with surgery; whereas, for pockets in excess of 4 mm, more gain in clinical attachment occurred following periodontal surgery by replaced flap, than following scaling and root planing.[8,9] These results confirm the favourable results after surgical elimination of deeper pockets.

Following periodontal surgery, maintenance by regular plaque control is essential. This should be monitored by the clinician, with reinforcement where necessary.[10] The frequency of recall needed by a patient can best be estimated by comparing the most recent plaque charts, the values on which help to determine the required period between professional help with preventive measures.

Given effective long-term postoperative care, studies have shown that the results of surgery are predictably good, with resolution of inflammation, stabilisation of the probing attachment level often at a more coronal position, and some deposition of new bone in osseous defects.[11,12] Patients who are not recalled regularly for monitoring and reinforcement of plaque control, generally show rapid deterioration of the periodontal condition with inflammation, recurrence of pocketing, and loss of probing attachment.[3,13,14] These studies emphasise the need to achieve sustained excellent oral hygiene before considering periodontal surgery, and the need to maintain this with professional help subsequent to surgical treatment. The frequency of recall visits is decided on the basis of the present plaque levels and the time elapsed since the last maintenance visit.

Management of the surgical patient

Preparation of the patient

It is essential that patients are fully informed about the aims and objectives of the operation before surgery. They must also be warned about any disadvantages which can be anticipated, for example, the likelihood of subsequent recession and the possibility of hypersensitivity to heat and to cold. The latter is generally only a temporary phenomenon provided that plaque control is maintained.

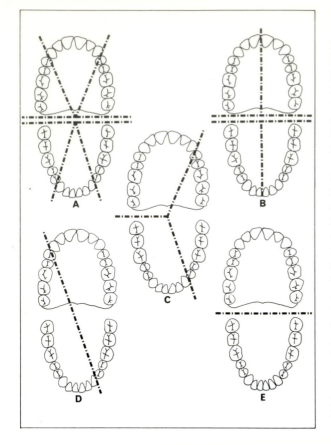

The operative procedure

Periodontal surgery is generally carried out under local analgesia. For the apprehensive patient, this may be augmented with intravenous sedation or relative analgesia. Where handicapped patients are to be treated, or where it is planned to undertake surgery on extensive areas at one visit, then hospitalisation and the use of general anaesthesia may be indicated.

Periodontal surgery is usually planned so that the mouth can be treated in segments, allowing one region to heal before progressing to the next. This enables the operator to decide the extent of the area to be undertaken at one visit, according to the complexity of the procedure. Other factors will also influence the planning of surgery, including the experience of the operator and the requirements of the patient. The use of sedation or general anaesthesia may enable a larger area to be undertaken or, perhaps, all the treatment to be completed at one session. It is comparatively rare for a patient after completion of plaque control treatment to require periodontal surgery involving all the teeth.

The patient should be given instructions about postoperative care. These are given verbally but may be reinforced by printed instructions.

POSTOPERATIVE ADVICE

Instructions for the week following periodontal surgery

1 If you have pain following periodontal surgery, take analgesic tablets such as paracetamol or aspirin in the dose advised by the manufacturer. If the pain persists or is severe, telephone for advice.

2 You may have had antibiotics prescribed; if so, you should take these as directed until the course of antibiotics has been completed.

3 If dressings have been applied these should remain in place until your next appointment. If any of the dressing comes away during the first two days or if the exposed area is painful or bleeds, you should telephone for advice.

4 There may be a minor amount of bleeding from the surgical site for the first day, but this should soon stop. Persistence of bleeding is uncommon, but can usually be controlled by the application of firm pressure to the area with a finger covered with a few layers of gauze or similar material. If the bleeding is severe or persists, or if there is undue swelling, you should telephone for advice.

5 Clean the unoperated regions of your mouth as usual.

6 The surgically treated area should be cleaned with a mouthwash. A salt solution may be used — add two teaspoonfuls of salt to half a glass of water. Alternatively you may have been advised to use an antiseptic mouthwash.

7 Strenuous exercise, smoking and alcohol should be avoided for the first few days after surgery. Avoid eating hard, spicy or sticky foods during the week after surgery. Try to avoid eating on teeth in the operated area.

Care during the second week after surgery

1 In those areas of the mouth which have not been treated surgically, use your normal cleaning methods.

2 Clean the surgical area both with the tooth-brush and between the teeth, using the methods you have been shown but with slightly less force to avoid damaging the healing gum.

3 Use a mouthwash if one has been prescribed.

Long-term care

1 Within about two weeks after surgery, cleaning procedures should be resumed using the normal amount of pressure. Both tooth-brushing and cleaning between the teeth must be performed thoroughly, and this routine must be continued in the future.

2 Attend your dentist regularly for routine examination and care. Regular assessment is essential to make sure that the inflammation of the gum does not recur.

Appendix 9
INSTRUMENTATION FOR PERIODONTAL SURGERY

It is convenient to assemble the basic instruments for periodontal surgery as a standardised kit which, after sterilisation, can be stored ready for use. The kit should be designed to contain those instruments used for more routine surgical procedures. It is advisable to cover with sterile material those parts of the equipment that the clinician may touch.

Contents of surgical tray

Towel clip
Sterile aluminium foil for operating light handle
Mirrors (2)
Probe no. 6 right angle
Probe—pocket measuring
College tweezers
Syringe for local analgesia
Aspirator tips
Tray for swabs
Scalpel handles (2)
Periosteal elevator—double-ended
Bowl for saline solution
Artery forceps—curved
Cumine scaler or similar
Excavator 125/126
Curettes for soft tissue and root planing (2)
Hoes (4)
Sharpening stone
Needle holders
Suture scissors
Tissue forceps
Ward's carver

Instruments which are used less frequently may be kept separately in individual sterile containers, thus avoiding too large or too many surgical kits.

Optional instruments - separately packed

Ultrasonic scaler tip
Bone chisels and files, e.g. Ochsenbein or Rhodes
Gingivectomy knives, e.g. Blake or Kirkland
Handpieces—straight or right-angled
Sterile burs

There are a number of accessory items

Consent form (if applicable)
Masks (2)
Safety glasses for operator, nurse and patient
Petroleum jelly
Topical anaesthetic
Local analgesic needles
Local analgesic cartridges
Hand towels
Gowns (2)
Surgical gloves (2 pairs)
Drapes for patient
Swabs
Saline
Disposable 20 ml syringe and needle
Periodontal dressing
Spatula
Sharps bin
Written postoperative instructions for patient
Analgesic tablets
Antiseptic mouthwash

OTHER TYPES OF SURGICAL INSTRUMENT

Periodontal surgery is generally carried out using conventional sharp-edged cutting instruments; several alternative techniques have been described, however, such as electrosurgery, cryosurgery and laser surgery.

Electrosurgery

To avoid detrimental effects it is necessary to control electrosurgical techniques carefully.[1] Waveform, frequency of alternation of the current, size of electrode, duration of the cutting radiation and the period for cooling between repeated cuts are all critical. A high frequency unit turned to optimal power output should be used with a fully filtered rectified waveform. A small electrode should be used and this should be kept moving through the tissue at a minimum of 7 mm per second. If reattachment of connective tissue is required, contact of the electrode with cementum must be avoided. Extended contact of the electrode with bone or incorrect current control may produce bone damage. Contact with metallic restorations for over 0.4 second may result in necrosis of the pulp.[1] The advantage of the procedure is mainly haemorrhage control, enabling restorative procedures to be undertaken immediately after surgery with a relatively blood-free field. The disadvantages include the expense of the equipment and the possibility of damage being caused by incorrect techniques. Several papers have described greater bone damage and delays in healing and remodelling after electrosurgery compared with conventional surgery.[2]

Cryosurgery

The technique of cryosurgery has been used in oral surgery procedures, for example, to reduce the size of vascular lesions enabling them to be excised subsequently with reduced risk of haemorrhage. No clear advantages have been reported for periodontal applications of the technique, the effect of the procedure being mainly on the superficial layers of the tissue. The procedure was found to be time-consuming, taking 2 applications of the tip at $-65°C$ for periods of 1 minute each to treat an area of 0.5 mm. The effect on the deeper tissues, for example the pocket epithelium, was minimal.[3]

Laser

The CO_2 laser has been used for periodontal treatment. The energy beam is produced by light amplification by stimulated emission of radiation. Photons reflected off mirrors in the reflective system collide with atoms that are already in an excited state, releasing still further photons and amplifying the radiation power. The photons produced by stimulated emissions all have the same velocity and direction, resulting in a rectilinear beam. The spectrum of the CO_2 laser beam coincides with the absorption spectrum of water and, at the focus of the beam, energy is released. This results in local destruction of soft tissue because of its high water content. The main advantage of the technique is the haemostatic effect. At present, the equipment is expensive and bulky; eye protection is essential for the operator, the assistant and the patient.[4] Satisfactory results have been reported after using laser surgery to remove hyperplastic gingiva.[5]

Appendix 10
PERIODONTAL BONE DEFECTS

ASSESSMENT

On completion of curettage and root planing, the alveolar bone is assessed to determine whether bone defects are present. If so, a thorough examination is necessary to check various associated factors, including the amount of bone support, the degree of mobility and the anatomical morphology of the region, for example the influence of a shallow palatal vault in the maxilla or of a wide ledge on the buccal aspect in the mandibular molar region as a result of the external oblique ridge. The teeth are then assessed individually to determine the degree of mobility, the length and shape of the roots, the presence of grooves or concavities in the root surfaces and in the posterior segments, the influence of radicular furcations.

CLASSIFICATION OF BONE DEFECTS

The bone defects are examined in detail and can be classified as shown in the following diagrams.

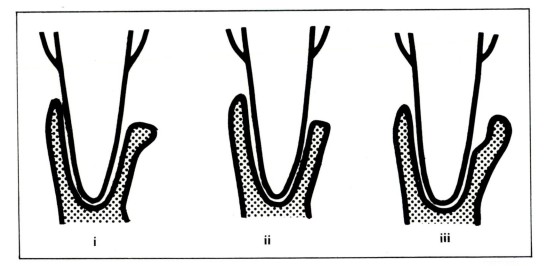

Exostoses, ledging and ditching. Marginal exostoses (i) may be caused by an alteration in the balance between bone resorption and bone deposition as a result of chronic inflammation. Ledging (ii) of the marginal bone results when there is a loss in height of bone without an accompanying reduction in thickness. Ditching (iii) is a type of one-walled defect and may involve several aspects of the tooth.

Reverse architecture and furcation involvement. (i) Reverse architecture results when there is a more rapid rate of resorption of the interproximal bone than marginal bone. (ii) On multirooted teeth bone loss from periodontal disease may result in exposure of the furcation regions.

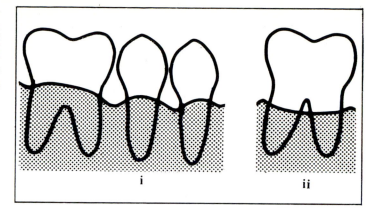

Three-, two- and one-walled defects. Infra-bony defects are classified by the number of bony walls present. The three-walled defect is illustrated in (i); the two-walled defect appears as in (ii) or alternatively as a crater (iii). The one-walled defect may occur as in (iv) or alternatively as a hemi-septal defect as in (v). Frequently the anatomy of bony defects is complicated. They may involve several aspects of the tooth, and may begin as three-walled, becoming two-walled and finally end as one-walled defects at their coronal extremity.

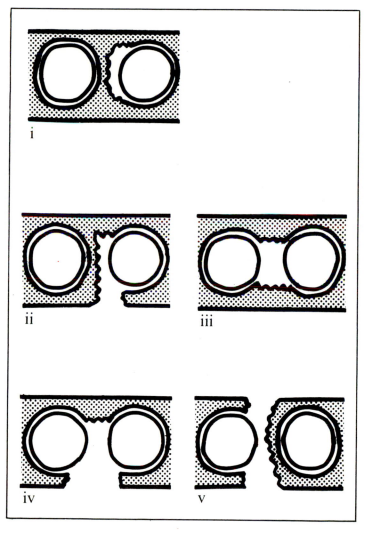

Appendix 11
PERIODONTAL SUTURING TECHNIQUES

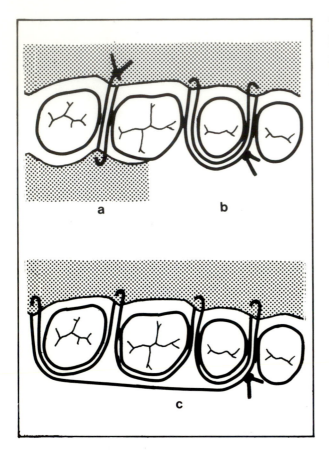

The objectives of interproximal suturing are to prevent the flap being displaced and to obtain adaptation of the flap to the underlying tissues. (a) Interrupted sutures are used when it is required to secure the buccal and palatal papillae under equal tension across the interproximal spaces. (b) The sling suture is used to suspend adjoining papillae without involving the papillae on the opposite aspect of the teeth. (c) The continuous suture is used to suspend the papillae of several consecutive teeth. It can be used for securing a buccal flap which has been used in conjunction with a palatal gingivectomy. The continuous suture is also useful for securing buccal and palatal flaps under independent tensions. For example, the buccal flap may be sutured relatively loosely to permit it to be repositioned apically. The palatal flap which is to be replaced is then sutured under slight tension.

The flap must also be stabilised against movement in a coronal direction. The position of the flap at the relieving incision is determined by the placement of the lateral suture (375). Maximum apical movement is achieved by placing the suture through the papilla on the flap and at the muco-gingival junction on the unoperated tissue. Where there is difficulty in maintaining the flap in the correct relationship, a periosteal suture may be used. The suture is passed through the mucosa of the vestibule and into the underlying periosteum. It is then brought out again through the mucosa and tied. This is a difficult technique and in some regions of the mouth the periosteum is not thick enough to permit a suture to be placed.

The most common method of providing resistance to coronal movement of the flap is by careful placement of a periodontal dressing. For a repositioned flap, the material should be of firm consistency when placed so that it has sufficient body to control the flap. Retention of the dressing is obtained by applying pressure over each interproximal region to obtain adaptation.

Appendix 12
WOUND HEALING

Wound healing after periodontal treatment may occur by any of the following responses:[1]

(a) **Repair**—healing of a wound by tissue that does not fully restore the architecture or the function of the part, for example, the formation of a long junctional epithelial attachment. Cells that have proliferated from the epithelial margins of the flap attach to the tooth by means of hemidesmosomes and a basal lamina. The length of this attachment may extend for several millimetres, and studies have shown that it is relatively stable.[2] It must be emphasised that, as with the follow-up of all periodontal procedures, stability of the attachment level in the long term is dependent on the maintenance of plaque control.

(b) **Reattachment**—the reunion of connective tissue with a root surface on which viable periodontal tissue has been retained. Procedures to retain the gingival fibres have been described.[3,4,5] One technique involves the use of an intracrevicular incision through to the bone. The incision leaves severed gingival fibres attached to cementum when the flap is elevated. Subsequently, root planing is restricted to the contaminated cementum surfaces, the retained gingival fibres being left intact. It has been shown in experimental studies that these severed fibres participate in forming a reattachment with the corium of the flap.

(c) **New attachment**—the reunion of connective tissue with a root surface that has been deprived of its periodontal ligament (for example, the formation of new cementum with inserting collagen fibres). In proximity to the periodontal ligament, cells from this source proliferate and migrate coronally. Cells from the ligament have the potential to form new cementum, even on root surfaces denuded of fibres. New periodontal and gingival fibres are inserted into this layer of cementum.[6] The extent of this migration of periodontal ligament cells is usually restricted to about 0.5 to 1 mm, although current research is investigating methods to extend this zone of new attachment.

(d) **Regeneration**—the reconstitution of the architecture and function of a lost or injured part (for example, ideal healing with all tissues being restored). Research has shown that regeneration is difficult to achieve, although work is continuing in this field.[7]

Maturation with formation of new sulcus

During the later stages of healing, maturation of the tissues occurs with the re-establishment of anatomical form. At this stage a new gingival sulcus is formed.

Summary

The surgical treatment of periodontal disease is designed to achieve reduction in pocketing; this may be by excision of excess tissue. The more conservative procedures aim to retain tissue and to treat the pocket, to obtain reduction in depth by soft tissue shrinkage, and by attachment of the soft tissues. Attachment may be achieved by a long junctional epithelial attachment, by reattachment, by new attachment or by regeneration.

Gingivectomy (see Chapter 11)

(a) The first stage in healing after gingivectomy is the formation of a blood clot over the wound surface.

(b) During the first 2 weeks after surgery granulation tissue forms within the clot, and epithelium from the wound edges migrates over this granulation tissue.

(c) From about day 10 to about day 30 there is organisation of connective tissue and keratinisation of epithelium. During this period a new junctional epithelium and gingival sulcus develop.[8]

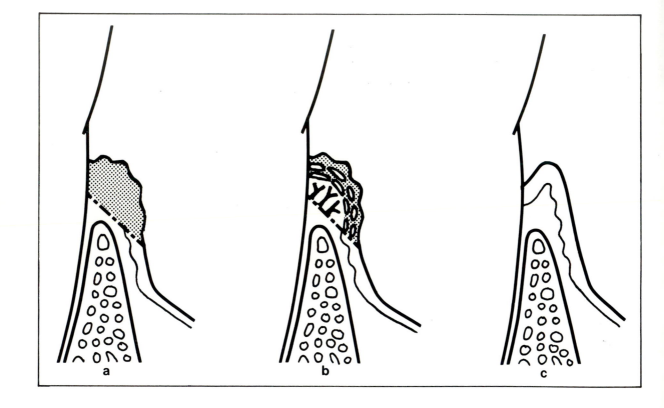

Periodontal flap surgery (see Chapter 12)

(a) The initial phase in the healing process after periodontal flap surgery is clot formation between the flap and the underlying tissue.

(b) In the first 2 weeks postoperatively granulation tissue develops within the clot. Near the surface of the clot, the space between the flap and the tooth is rapidly bridged by the migration of epithelial cells.

(b) and (c) The exposure of alveolar bone at the time of flap surgery results in subsequent resorption; this takes place mainly during the first 3 weeks after the operation.

The amount of net bone loss depends on several factors, for example, on the thickness of the marginal bone, on whether bone surgery is performed, and on whether the alveolar bone is completely covered with the flap after surgery, or whether a width of marginal bone is left exposed. Studies on human subjects indicate that there is a loss of 0.5 to 1 mm when bone is covered.[9] At the other extreme, there is severe and prolonged resorption of bone following denudation procedures in which bone is left exposed after surgery.[10]

(d) Towards the end of the initial 3-week period, deposition of bone begins and this continues for 10 weeks or more after surgery. As a result, there is a partial restoration of the lost bone.[11]

The organisation of the connective tissue, and the formation of a long junctional epithelial attachment and a gingival sulcus take place between approximately day 10 and day 40.

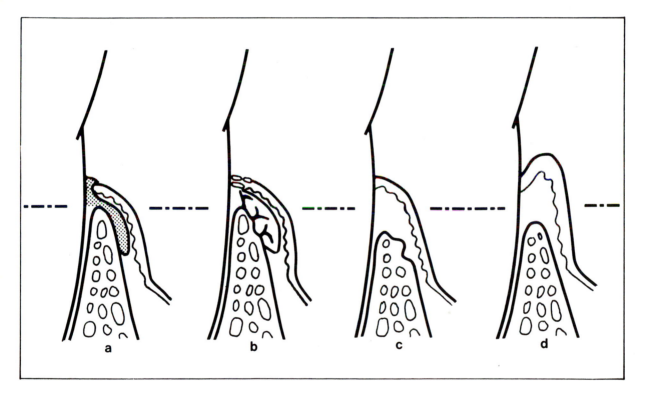

Bibliography

CHAPTER 1

1. Gaengler, P. and Merte, K. (1983). Effects of force application on periodontal blood circulation. *J. Periodont. Res.*, **18**, 86.

2. Weekes, W.T. and Sims, M.R. (1986). The vasculature of the rat molar gingival crevice. *J. Periodont. Res.*, **21**, 177.

3. Sims, M.R. (1978). Oxytalan fibre response to tooth intrusion and extrusion in normal and lathyritic mice. *J. Periodont. Res.*, **13**, 199.

4. Davies, R.M., Downer, M.C., Hull, P.S. and Lennon, M.A. (1974). Alveolar defects in human skulls. *J. Clin. Periodont.*, **1**, 107.

5. Edel, A. (1981). Alveolar bone fenestrations and dehiscences in dry Bedouin jaws. *J. Clin. Periodont.*, **8**, 491.

6. Lost, C. (1984). Depth of alveolar bone dehiscences in relation to gingival recessions. *J. Clin. Periodont.*, **11**, 583.

7. Listgarten, M.A. (1972). Gingival Epithelium. *Oral Sciences Review* 1. Munksgaard Publishers. Copenhagen.

8. Listgarten, M.A. (1980). Periodontal probing: what does it mean? *J. Clin. Periodont.*, **7**, 165.

9. Fowler, C., Garrett, S., Crigger, M. and Egelberg, J. (1982). Histologic probe position in treated and untreated human periodontal tissues. *J. Clin. Periodont.*, **9**, 373.

10. Stern, I.B. (1981). Current concepts of the dentogingival junction: the epithelial and connective tissue attachments to the tooth. *J. Periodontol.*, **52**, 465.

11. Melcher, A.H. and Eastoe, J.E. (1969). *Biology of the Periodontium*. Academic Press. London, New York.

12. Folke, L.E.A. and Stallard, R.E. (1967). Periodontal microcirculation as revealed by plastic microspheres. *J. Periodont. Res.*, **2**, 53.

13. Hock, J. (1975). Gingival vasculature around erupting deciduous teeth of dogs and cats. *J. Clin. Periodont.*, **2**, 44.

14. Karring, T., Ostergaard, G.E. and Loe, H. (1971). Conservation of tissue specificity after heterotopic transplantation of gingiva and alveolar mucosa. *J. Periodont. Res.*, **6**, 282.

15. Karring, T., Cumming, B.R., Oliver, R.C. and Loe, H. (1975). The origin of granulation tissue and its impact on postoperative results of mucogingival surgery. *J. Periodontol.*, **46**, 577.

16. Bakdash, B.M., Jernberg, G.R. and Keenan, K.M. (1983). Relationship between proximal tooth open contacts and periodontal disease. *J. Periodontol.*, **54**, 529.

17. Bowers, G.M. (1963). A study of the width of attached gingiva. *J. Periodontol.*, **34**, 201.

18. Lang, N.P. and Loe, H. (1972). The relationship between width of keratinized gingiva and gingival health. *J. Periodontol.*, **43**, 623.

19. Miyasato, M., Crigger, M. and Egelberg, J. (1977). Gingival condition in areas of minimal and appreciable width of keratinized gingiva. *J. Clin. Periodont.*, **4**, 200.

20. Wennstrom, J. and Lindhe, J. (1983). Role of attached gingiva for maintenance of periodontal health. *J. Clin. Periodont.*, **10**, 206.

21. Kisch, J., Badersten, A. and Egelberg, J. (1986). Longitudinal observation of 'unattached', mobile gingival areas. *J. Clin. Periodont.*, **13**, 131.

22. Powell, R.N. and McEniery, T.M. (1982). A longitudinal study of isolated gingival recession in the mandibular central incisor region of children aged 6-8 years. *J. Clin. Periodont.*, **9**, 357.

23. Smukler, H. and Machtei, E. (1987). Gingival recession and plaque control. *Compend. Contin. Educ. Dent.*, **8**, 194.

24. Withers, J.A., Brunsvold, M.A., Killoy, W.J. and Rahe, A.J. (1981). The relationship of palato-gingival grooves to localised periodontal disease. *J. Periodontol.*, **52**, 41.

25. Kogon, S.L. (1986). The prevalence, location and conformation of palato-radicular grooves in maxillary incisors. *J. Periodontol.*, **57**, 231.

CHAPTER 2

1. Theilade, E., Wright, W.H., Jensen, S.B. and Loe, H. (1966). Experimental gingivitis in man II. A longitudinal clinical and bacteriological investigation. *J. Periodont. Res.*, **1**, 1.

2. Gibbons, R.J. and van Houte, J. (1973). On the formation of dental plaques. *J. Periodontol.*, **44**, 347.

3. Kornman, K.S. (1986). The role of supragingival plaque in the prevention and treatment of periodontal diseases. A review of current concepts. *J. Periodont. Res.*, **21**, Supplement 5.

4. Moore, W.E., Holdeman, L.V., Smibert, R.M., Good, I.J., Burmeister, J.A., Palcanis, K.G. and Ranney, R.R. (1982). Bacteriology of experimental gingivitis in young adult humans. *Infection and Immunity*, **38**, 651.

5. Listgarten, M.A. (1987). Nature of periodontal diseases: pathogenic mechanisms. *J. Periodont. Res.*, **22**, 172.

6. Loe, H., Theilade, E. and Jensen, S.B. (1965). Experimental gingivitis in man. *J. Periodontol.*, **36**, 177.

7. Van Palenstein Helderman, W.H. (1986). Is antibiotic therapy justified in the treatment of human chronic inflammatory periodontal disease? *J. Clin. Periodont.*, **13**, 932.

8. Slots, J. (1986). Bacterial specificity in adult periodontitis. *J. Clin. Periodont.*, **13**, 912.

9. Page, R.C. (1986). Gingivitis. *J. Clin. Periodont.*, **13**, 345.

10. Slots, J. and Listgarten, M.A. (1988). *Bacteroides gingivalis*, *Bacteroides intermedius* and *Actinobacillus actinomycetemcomitans* in human periodontal diseases. *J. Clin Periodont.*, **15**, 85.

11. Listgarten, M.A. (1988). A rationale for monitoring the periodontal microbiota after periodontal treatment. *J. Periodontol.*, **59**, 439.

12. Listgarten, M.A. (1988). The role of dental plaque in gingivitis and periodontitis. *J. Clin. Periodont.*, **15**, 485.

13. Dzink, J.L., Tanner, A.C.R., Haffajee, A.D. and Socransky, S.D. (1985). Gram negative species associated with active destructive periodontal lesions. *J. Clin. Periodont.*, **12**, 648.

14. Dzink, J.L., Socransky, S.S. and Haffajee, A.D. (1988). The predominant cultivable microbiota of active and inactive lesions of destructive periodontal diseases. *J. Clin. Periodont.*, **15**, 316.

15. Goodson, J.M., Haffajee, A.D. and Socransky, S.S. (1984). The relationship between attachment level loss and alveolar bone loss. *J. Clin. Periodont.*, **11**, 348.

16. Clerehugh, V. and Lennon, M.A. (1986). The radiographic measurement of early periodontal bone loss and its relationship with clinical loss of attachment. *Br. Dent. J.*, **161**, 141.

17. Romanowski, A.W., Squier, C.A. and Lesch, C.A. (1988). Permeability of rodent junctional epithelium to exogenous protein. *J. Periodont. Res.*, **23**, 81.

18. Seymour, G.J., Powell, R.N. and Davies, W.I.R., (1979). Conversion of a stable T-cell lesion to a progressive B-cell lesion in the pathogenesis of chronic inflammatory periodontal disease — an hypothesis. *J. Clin. Periodont.*, **6**, 267.

19. Schroeder, H.E. and Lindhe, J. (1980). Conditions and pathological features of rapidly destructive, experimental periodontitis in dogs. *J. Periodontol.*, **51**, 6.

20. Sanavi, F., Listgarten, M.A., Boyd, F., Sallay, K. and Nowotny, A. (1985). The colonization and establishment of invading bacteria in periodontium of ligature-treated immunosuppressed rats. *J. Periodontol.*, **56**, 273.

21. Saglie, F.R., Carranza, F.A. and Newman, M.G. (1985). The presence of bacteria within the oral epithelium in periodontal disease — I. Scanning and transmission electron microscopic study. *J. Periodontol.*, **56**, 618.

22. Page, R.C. and Schroeder, H.E. (1976). Pathogenesis of inflammatory periodontal disease. A summary of current work. *Laboratory Investigations*, **33**, 235.

23. Schluger, S., Youdelis, R.A. and Page, R.C. (1978). *Periodontal Disease*. Lea & Febiger. U.S.A.

24. Sterrett J.D. (1986). The osteoclast and periodontitis. *J. Clin. Periodont.*, **13**, 258.

25. Lindemann, R.A. and Economou, J.S. (1988). *Actinobacillus actinomycetemcomitans* and *Bacteroides gingivalis* activate human peripheral monocytes to produce interleukin-1 and tumor necrosis factor. *J. Periodontol.*, **59**, 728.

26. Mukherjee, S. (1968). Formation and prevention of supra-gingival calculus. *J. Periodont. Res.*, Supplement No. 2.

27. Mandel, I.D. and Gaffar, A. (1986). Calculus revisited. A review. *J. Clin. Periodont.*, **13**, 249.

28. Pennel, B.M. and Keagle, J.G. (1977). Predisposing factors in the aetiology of chronic inflammatory periodontal disease. *J. Periodontol.*, **48**, 524.

29. Gorzo, I., Newman, H.N. and Strahan, J.D. (1979). Amalgam restorations, plaque removal and periodontal health. *J. Clin. Periodont.*, **6**, 98.

30. Bergman, B., Hugoson, A. and Olsson, C. (1971). Periodontal and prosthetic conditions in patients treated with removable partial dentures and artificial crowns. A longitudinal 2-year study. *Acta. Odontol. Scand.*, **29**, 621.

31. Kratchovil, F.J., Davidson, P.N. and Guijt, J. (1982). Five-year survey of treatment with removable partial dentures, Part 1. *J. Prosth. Dent.*, **48**, 237.

32. Addy, M., Dummer P.M.H., Hunter, M.L., Kingdon, A. and Shaws, W.C. (1987). A study of the association of fraenal attachment, lip coverage, and vestibular depth with plaque and gingivitis. *J. Periodontol.*, **58**, 752.

33. Rivera-Hidalgo, F. (1986). Smoking and periodontal disease, a review of the literature. *J. Periodontol.*, **57**, 617.

34. Baab, D.A. and Oberg, P.A. (1987). The effect of cigarette smoking on gingival blood flow in humans. *J. Clin. Periodont.*, **14**, 418.

CHAPTER 3

1. Johnson, N.W., Griffiths, G.S., Wilton, J.M.A., Maiden, M.F.J., Curtis, M.A., Gillett, I.R., Wilson, D.T. and Sterne, J.A.C. (1988). Detection of high-risk groups and individuals for periodontal diseases. *J. Clin. Periodont.*, **15**, 276.

2. Page, R.C., Altman, L.C., Ebersole, J.L., Vandsteen, G.E., Dahlberg, W.H., Williams, B.L. and Osterberg, S.K. (1983). Rapidly progressive periodontitis, a distinct clinical condition. *J. Periodontol.*, **54**, 197.

3. Baer, P.N. (1971). The case for periodontosis as a clinical entity. *J. Periodontol.*, **42**, 516.

4. Page, R.C., Vandesteen, G.E., Ebersole, J.L., Williams, B.L., Dixon, E.I. and Altman, L.C. (1985). Clinical and laboratory studies of a family with a high prevalence of juvenile periodontitis. *J. Periodontol.*, **56**, 602.

5. Kaslick, R.S., West, T.L. and Chasesens, A.I. (1980). Association between ABO blood groups, HL-A antigens and periodontal diseases in young adults. *J. Periodontol.*, **51**, 339.

6. Saxen, L. and Koskimies, S. (1984). Juvenile periodontitis - no linkage with HLA-antigens. *J. Periodont. Res.*, **19**, 441.

7. Saxen, L. (1980). Juvenile periodontitis. *J. Clin. Periodont.*, **7**, 1.

8. Davies, R.M., Smith, R.G. and Porter, S.R. (1985). Destructive forms of periodontal disease in adolescents and young adults. *Br. Dent. J.*, **158**, 429.

9. Saxby, M.A. (1987). Juvenile periodontitis: an epidemiological study in the West Midlands of the United Kingdom. *J. Clin. Periodont.*, **14**, 594.

10. Hormand, J. and Frandsen, A. (1979). Juvenile periodontitis. Localization of bone loss in relation to age, sex and teeth. *J. Clin. Periodont.*, **6**, 407.

11. Saxen, L. and Murtomaa, H. (1985). Age-related expression of juvenile periodontitis. *J. Clin. Periodont.*, **12**, 21.

12. Ellegaard, B., Borregaard, N. and Ellegaard, J. (1984). Neutrophil chemotaxis and phagocytosis in juvenile periodontitis. *J. Periodont. Res.*, **19**, 261.

13. Sandholm, L. (1985). The cellular host response in juvenile periodontitis. *J. Periodontol.*, **56**, 539.

14. Van Dyke, T.E., Schweinebraten M., Cianciola, L.J., Offenbacher, S. and Genco, R.J. (1985). Neutrophil chemotaxis in families with localized juvenile periodontitis. *J. Periodont. Res.*, **20**, 503.

15. Liljenberg, B. and Lindhe, J. (1980). Juvenile periodontitis. Some microbiological, histopathological and clinical characteristics. *J. Clin. Periodont.*, **7**, 48.

16. Baab, D.A., Page, R.C. Ebersole, J.L., Williams, B.L. and Scott C.R. (1986). Laboratory studies of a family manifesting premature exfoliation of deciduous teeth. *J. Clin. Periodont.*, **13**, 677.

17. Ebersole, J.L., Haffajee, A.D., Smith, D.J. and Socransky, S.S. (1984). Clinical, microbiological and immunological features associated with the treatment of active periodontosis lesions. *J. Clin. Periodont.*, **11**, 600.

18. Zambon, J.J. (1985). *Actinobacillus actinomycetemcomitans* in human periodontal disease. *J. Clin. Periodont.*, **12**, 1.

19. Tsai, C.C. and Taichman, S. (1986). Dynamics of infection by leukotoxic strains of *Actinobacillus actinomycetemcomitans* in juvenile periodontitis. *J. Clin. Periodont.*, **11**, 330.

20. Waerhaug, J. (1977). Plaque control in the treatment of juvenile periodontitis. *J. Clin. Periodont.*, **4**, 29.

21. Hoffman, I.D. (1983). Familial occurrence of juvenile periodontitis with varied treatment of one of the siblings with five-year follow-up. *J. Periodontol.*, **54**, 44.

22. Gillett, R. and Johnson, N.W. (1982). Bacterial invasion of the periodontium in a case of juvenile periodontitis. *J. Clin. Periodont.*, **9**, 93.

23. Lindhe, J. and Liljenberg, B. (1984). Treatment of localized juvenile periodontitis. Results after 5 years. *J. Clin. Periodont.*, **11**, 399.

24. Rosling, B.G. and Slots, J. (1983). Suppression of the periodontopathic microflora in localized juvenile periodontitis by systemic tetracycline. *J. Clin. Periodont.*, **10**, 465.

25. Christersson, L.A., Slots, J., Rosling, B.G. and Genco, R.J. (1985). Microbiological and clinical effects of surgical treatment of localized juvenile periodontitis. *J. Clin. Periodont.*, **12**, 465.

26. Mandell, R.L., Tripodi, L.S., Savitt, E., Goodson, J.M. and Socransky, S.S. (1986). The effect of treatment on *Actinobacillus actinomycetemcomitans* in localized juvenile periodontitis. *J. Periodontol.*, **57**, 94.

27. Murro, C.D., Nisini, R., Cattabriga, M., Simonetti-D'Arca, A., Le Moli, S., Paolantonio, M., Sebastiani, L. and D'Amelio, R. (1987). Neutrophil chemotaxis inhibitory factors associated with the presence of *Bacteroides gingivalis* in crevicular fluid. *J. Periodontol.*, **58**, 868.

28. Hirschfeld, L. and Wasserman, B. (1978). A long-term survey of tooth loss in 600 treated periodontal patients. *J. Periodontol.*, **49**, 225.

29. Lindhe, J. and Nyman, S. (1984). Long-term maintenance of patients treated for advanced periodontal disease. *J. Clin. Periodont.*, **11**, 504.

30. Goldman, M.J., Ross, I.F. and Goteiner, D. (1986). Effect of periodontal therapy on patients maintained for 15 years or longer. *J. Periodontol.*, **57**, 347.

31. Lundstrom, A., Johansson, L.A. and Hamp, S.E. (1984). Effect of combined systemic antimicrobial therapy and mechanical plaque control in patients with recurrent periodontal disease. *J. Clin. Periodont.*, **11**, 321.

32. Bragd, L., Dahlen, G., Wikstrom, M. and Slots J. (1987). The capability of *Actinobacillus actinomycetemcomitans*, *Bacteroides gingivalis* and *Bacteroides intermedius* to indicate progressive periodontitis; a retrospective study. *J. Clin. Periodont.*, **14**, 95.

CHAPTER 4

1. Saxen, L., Aula, S. and Westermark, T. (1977). Periodontal disease associated with Down's syndrome. An orthopantomographic evaluation. *J. Periodontol.*, **48**, 337.

2. Saxen, L. and Aula, S. (1982). Periodontal bone loss in patients with Down's syndrome: a follow-up study. *J. Periodontol.*, **53**, 158.

3. Brown, R.H. (1978). A longitudinal study of periodontal disease in Down's syndrome. *N.Z. Dent. J.*, **74**, 137.

4. Reuland-Bosma, W., Van Dijk, L.J. and Van der Weele, L. (1986). Experimental gingivitis around deciduous teeth in children with Down's syndrome. *J. Clin. Periodont.*, **13**, 294.

5. Scully, C. (1976). Down's syndrome: aspects of dental care. *J. Dent.*, **4**, 167.

6. Baghadi, V.S. (1982). Papillon-Lefevre syndrome: report of four cases. *J. Dent. Child.*, **49**, 147.

7. Jung, J., Carranza, F.A., and Newman, M.G. (1981). Scanning electron-microscopy of plaque in Papillon-Lefevre syndrome. *J. Periodontol.*, **52**, 442.

8. Lyberg, T. (1982). Immunological and metabolical studies in two siblings with Papillon-Lefevre syndrome. *J. Periodont. Res.*, **17**, 563.

9. Jenkins, W.M.M., Murray, J.J., Sloan, P. and Soames, J.V. (1984). Histopathological and ultrastructural findings in a case of Papillon-Lefevre syndrome. *J. Periodontol.*, **55**, 482.

10. Munford, A.G. (1976). Papillon-Lefevre Syndrome. Report of two cases in the same family. *J. Am. Dent. Assoc.*, **93**, 121.

11. Sutcliffe, P. (1972). A longitudinal study of gingivitis and puberty. *J. Periodont. Res.*, 7, 52.

12. Loe, H. and Silness, J. (1963). Periodontal disease in pregnancy. *Acta. Odontol. Scand.*, 21, 533.

13. Cohen, D.W., Friedman, L., Shapiro, J. and Kyle, G. (1971). A longitudinal investigation of the periodontal changes during pregnancy II. *J. Periodontol.*, 42, 653.

14. Hugoson, A. (1970). Gingival inflammation and female sex hormones. *J. Periodont. Res.* Supplement No. 5.

15. Kornman, K.S. and Loesche, W.J. (1980). The subgingival microbial flora during pregnancy. *J. Periodont. Res.*, 15, 111.

16. Lindhe, J. and Bjorn, H. (1967). Influence of hormonal contraceptives on the gingiva of women. *J. Periodont. Res.*, 2, 1.

17. Nisengard, R.J., and Rogers, R.S. (1987). The treatment of desquamative gingival lesions. *J. Periodontol.*, 58, 167.

18. Cohen, D.W., Friedman, L.A., Shapiro, J., Kyle, G.C. and Franklin, S. (1970). Diabetes and periodontal disease: two year longitudinal observations. *J. Periodontol.*, 41, 709.

19. Rylander, H., Ramberg, P., Blohme, G. and Lindhe, J. (1986). Prevalence of periodontal disease in young diabetics. *J. Clin. Periodont.*, 14, 38.

20. McMullen, J.A., van Dyke, T.E., Horoszewicz, J.U. and Genco, R.J. (1981). Neutrophil chemotaxis in individuals with advanced periodontal disease and a genetic predisposition to diabetes mellitus. *J. Periodontol.*, 52, 167.

21. Frantzis, T.G., Reeve, C.M. and Brown, A.L. (1971). The ultrastructure of capillary basement membranes in the attached gingiva of diabetic and non-diabetic patients with periodontal disease. *J. Periodontol.*, 42, 406.

22. Barrett, A.P. (1984). Gingival lesions in leukemia. *J. Periodontol.*, 55, 585.

23. Barrett, A.P. (1987). Neutropenic ulceration. A distinctive clinical entity. *J. Periodontol.*, 58, 51.

24. Darby, W.J. (1979). Some observations concerning nutrition and dental health. *J. Clin. Periodont.*, 6, Extra Issue, 37.

25. Donnenfeld, O.W., Stanley, H.R. and Bagdonoff, L. (1974). A nine month clinical and histological study of patients on diphenylhydantoin following gingivectomy. *J. Periodontol.*, 45, 547.

26. Barak, S., Engelberg, I.S. and Hiss, J. (1986). Gingival hyperplasia caused by nifedipine. Histopathologic findings. *J. Periodontol.*, 58, 639.

27. Howell, L.P., Lucas, R.M. and Wall, B.A. (1985). Nifedipine-induced gingival hyperplasia. A histochemical and ultrastructural study. *J. Periodontol.*, 56, 211.

28. Daley, T.D. and Wysocki, G.P. (1984). Cyclosporin therapy. It's significance to the dentist. *J. Periodontol.*, 55, 708.

29. McGaw, T., Lam, S. and Coates, J. (1987). Cyclosporin-induced gingival overgrowth: correlation with dental plaque scores, gingivitis scores, and cyclosporin levels in serum and saliva. *Oral Surg., Oral Med. and Oral Path.*, 64, 293.

CHAPTER 5

1. Newman, M.G. and Sims, T.N., (1979). The predominant cultivable microbiota of the periodontal abscess. *J. Periodontol.*, 50, 350.

2. Peel, M.M., Rich, A.M. and Reade, P.C. (1981). *Actinobacillus actinomycetemcomitans* infection in the oral cavity. *Oral. Surg.*, 52, 591.

3. Harrington, G.W. (1979). The perio-endo question: differential diagnosis. *Dent. Clin. N. Am.*, 23, 673.

4. Epstein, S. and Scopp, I.W. (1977). Antibiotics and the intra-oral abscess. *J. Periodontol.*, 48, 236.

5. Miyasato, M.C. (1975). The periodontal abscess. *Periodontal Abstracts*, 23, 53.

6. Kareha, M.J., Rosenberg, E.S. and Dehaven, H. (1981). Therapeutic considerations in the management of a periodontal abscess with an intrabony defect. *J. Clin. Periodont.*, 8, 374.

7. Kowolik, M.J. and Nisbet, T. (1983). Smoking and acute ulcerative gingivitis. A study of 100 patients. *Br. Dent. J.*, 154, 241.

8. Loesche, W.J., Syed, S.A., Laughon, B.E. and Stoll, J. (1982). The bacteriology of acute necrotizing ulcerative gingivitis. Review. *J. Periodontol.*, 53, 223.

9. Falkler, W.A., Martin, S.A., Vincent, W., Tall, B.D., Nauman, R.K. and Suzuki, J.B. (1987). A clinical

demographic and microbiologic study of ANUG patients in an urban dental school. *J. Clin. Periodont.*, **14**, 307.

10. Cogen, R.B., Stevens, A.W., Cohen-Cole, S., Kirk, K. and Freeman, A. (1983). Leukocyte function in the etiology of acute necrotizing ulcerative gingivitis. *J. Periodontol.*, **54**, 402.

11. Listgarten, M.A. (1965). Electron microscope observation on the bacterial flora of acute necrotizing ulcerative gingivitis. *J. Periodontol.*, **36**, 328.

12. Duckworth, R., Waterhouse, J.P., Britton, D.E.R., Nuki, K., Sheiham, A., Winter, R. and Blake, G.C. (1966). A double-blind controlled clinical trial of metronidazole. *Br. Dent. J.*, **120**, 599.

13. Cawson, R.A. (1986). Update on antiviral chemotherapy: the advent of acyclovir. *Br. Dent. J.*, **161**, 245.

CHAPTER 6

1. Jandinski, J.J. and Shklar, G. (1976). Lichen planus of the gingiva. *J. Periodontol.*, **47**, 724.

2. Nisengard, R.J. and Neiders, M. (1981). Desquamative lesions of the gingiva. *J. Periodontol.*, **52**, 500.

3. Nisengard, R.J. and Rogers, R.S. (1987). The treatment of desquamative gingival lesions. *J. Periodontol.*, **58**, 167.

CHAPTER 7

1. Socransky, S.S. and Manganiello, S.D. (1971). The oral microbiota of man from birth to senility. *J. Periodontol.*, **42**, 485.

2. Longhurst, P., Johnson, N.W. and Hopps, R.M. (1977). Differences in lymphocyte and plasma cell densities in inflamed gingiva from adults and young children. *J. Periodontol.*, **48**, 705.

3. Matsson, L. and Goldberg, P. (1985). Gingival inflammatory reaction in children at different ages. *J. Clin. Periodont.*, **12**, 98.

4. Muhlemann, H.R. (1958). Gingivitis in Zurich schoolchildren. *Helv. Odont. Acta.*, **2**, 3.

5. Sutcliffe, P., (1972). A longitudinal study of gingivitis and puberty. *J. Periodont. Res.*, **7**, 52.

6. Yanover, L. and Ellen, R.P. (1986). A clinical and microbiologic examination of gingival disease in parapubescent females. *J. Periodontol.*, **57**, 562.

7. Wojcicki, C.J., Harper, D.S. and Robinson, P.J. (1987). Differences in periodontal disease-associated micro-organisms of subgingival plaque in prepubertal, pubertal and post-pubertal children. *J. Periodontol.*, **58**, 219.

8. Stamm, J.W. (1986). Epidemiology of gingivitis. *J. Clin. Periodont.*, **13**, 360.

9. Hull, P.S., Hillam, D.G. and Beal, J.F. (1975). A radiographic study of the prevalence of chronic periodontitis in 14-year-old English schoolchildren. *J. Clin. Periodont.*, **2**, 203.

10. Blankenstein, R., Murray, J.J. and Lind, O.P. (1978). Prevalence of chronic periodontitis in 13-15 year old children. *J. Clin. Periodont.*, **5**, 285.

11. Gjermo, P., Bellini, H.T., Santos, V.P., Martins, J.G. and Ferracyoli, J.R. (1984). Prevalence of bone loss in a group of Brazilian teenagers assessed on bite-wing radiographs. *J. Clin. Periodont.*, **11**, 104.

12. Hansen, B.F., Gjermo, P. and Larsen, K.R.B. (1984). Periodontal bone loss in 15-year old Norwegians. *J. Clin. Periodont.*, **11**, 125.

13. Clerehugh, V. and Lennon, M.A. (1986). The radiographic measurement of early periodontal bone loss and its relationship with clinical loss of attachment. *Br. Dent. J.*, **161**, 141.

14. Lennon, M.A. and Davies, R.M. (1974). Prevalence and distribution of alveolar bone loss in a population of 15 year old schoolchildren. *J. Clin. Periodont.*, **1**, 175.

15. Waite, I.M. and Furniss, J. (1987). Periodontal disease in children. *J. Paed. Dentistry*, **3**, 59.

16. Greene, J.C. and Vermillion, J.R. (1963). The effects of controlled oral hygiene on the human adult periodontium. *Int. Dent. J.*, **21**, 8.

17. Loe, H. Anerud, A., Boysen, H. and Smith, M. (1978). The natural history of periodontal disease in man. The rate of periodontal destruction before 40 years of age. *J. Periodontol.*, **49**, 607.

18. Miller, A.J., Brunelle, J.A., Carlos, J.P., Brown, L.J. and Loe, H (1987). *Oral health of United States adults. Epidemiology and oral disease prevention program.* U.S. Department of Health and Human Services. National Institute of Health Publication No. 87-2868.

19. Socransky, S.S., Haffajee, A.D., Goodson, J.M. and Lindhe, J. (1984). New concepts of destructive periodontal disease. *J. Clin. Periodont.*, **11**, 21.

20. Haffajee, A.D. and Socransky, S.S. (1986). Attachment level changes in destructive periodontal diseases. *J. Clin. Periodontol.*, **13**, 461.

21. Albandar, J.M., Rise, J., Gjermo, P. and Johansen, J.R. (1986). Radiographic quantification of alveolar bone level changes. A 2-year longitudinal study in man. *J. Clin. Periodont.*, **13**, 195.

22. Ralls, S.A. and Cohen, M.E. (1986). Problems in identifying "bursts" of periodontal attachment loss. *J. Periodontol.*, **57**, 746.

23. Lindhe, J., Haffajee, A.D. and Socransky, S.S. (1983). Progression of periodontal disease in adult subjects in the absence of periodontal therapy. *J. Clin. Periodont.*, **10**, 433.

24. Baelum, V., Fejerskov O. and Karring, T. (1986). Oral hygiene, gingivitis and periodontal breakdown in adult Tanzanians. *J. Periodont. Res.*, **21**, 221.

25. Loe, H., Anerud, A., Boysen, H. and Smith, M. (1978). The natural history of periodontal disease in man. Tooth mortality rates before 40 years of age. *J. Periodont. Res.*, **13**, 563.

26. Loe, H., Anerud, A., Boysen, H. and Morrison, E. (1986). Natural history of periodontal disease in man. Rapid, moderate and no loss of attachment in Sri-Lankan laborers 14 to 46 years of age. *J. Clin. Periodont.*, **13**, 431.

27. Baelum, V., Fejerskov, O. and Manji, F. (1988). Periodontal diseases in adult Kenyans. *J. Clin. Periodont.*, **15**, 445.

28. Reddy, J., Africa, C.W. and Parker, J.R. (1986). Darkfield microscopy of subgingival plaque of an urban black population with poor oral hygiene. *J. Clin. Periodont.*, **13**, 578.

29. Loe, H. (1988). Periodontics of tomorrow. *Dent. Clin. N. Amer.*, **32**, 395.

CHAPTER 8

1. Miller, S.C. (1950). *Textbook of Periodontia.* The Blakeston Co. Philadelphia.

2. Grant, D.A., Stern, I.B. and Listgarten, M.A. (1988). *Periodontics, Sixth Edition.* C.V. Mosby Company. St. Louis.

3. Van Der Velden, U. (1982). Location of probe tip in bleeding and non-bleeding pockets with minimal gingival inflammation. *J. Clin. Periodont.*, **9**, 421.

4. Caton, J., Thilo, B., Polson, A. and Espeland, M. (1988). Cell populations associated with conversion from bleeding to nonbleeding gingiva. *J. Periodontol.*, **59**, 7.

5. Aeppli, D.M., Boen, J.R. and Bandt, C.L. (1985). Measuring and interpreting increases in probing depth and attachment loss. *J. Periodontol.*, **56**, 262.

CHAPTER 9

1. O'Leary, T.J., Drake, R.B. and Naylor, J.E. (1972). The Plaque Control Record. *J. Periodontol.*, **43**, 38.

2. Tan, A.E.S. and Wade, A.B. (1980). The role of visual feedback by a disclosing agent in plaque control. *J. Clin. Periodont.*, **7**, 140.

3. Axelsson, P. and Lindhe, J. (1978). Effect of controlled oral hygiene procedures on caries and periodontal disease in adults. *J. Clin. Periodont.*, **5**, 133.

4. Axelsson, P. and Lindhe, J. (1981). The significance of maintenance care in the treatment of periodontal disease. *J. Clin. Periodont.*, **8**, 281.

5. Hodge, H.C., Holloway, P.J. and Bell, C.R. (1982). Factors associated with toothbrushing behaviour in adolescents. *Br. Dent. J.*, **152**, 49.

6. Wilson, T.G. (1986). Compliance — a review of the literature with possible implications to periodontics. *J. Periodontol.*, **58**, 706.

7. Smukler, H. and Landsberg, J. (1984). The toothbrush and gingival traumatic injury. *J. Periodontol.*, **55**, 713.

8. Bergenholtz, A. (1972). Mechanical cleaning in oral hygiene. *Oral Hygiene*. Munksgaard. Copenhagen.

9. Gjermo, P. and Flotra, L. (1970). The effect of different methods of interdental cleaning. *J. Periodont. Res.*, **5**, 230.

10. Wolfe, G.N. (1976). An evaluation of proximal surface cleansing agents. *J. Clin. Periodont.*, **3**, 148.

11. Lamberts, D.M., Wunderlich, R.C. and Cafesse, R.G. (1982). The effect of waxed and unwaxed dental floss on gingival health — Part I: plaque removal and gingival response. *J. Periodontol.*, **53**, 393.

12. Bergenholtz, A. and Brithon, J. (1980). Plaque removal by dental floss or toothpicks. An intra-individual comparative study. *J. Clin. Periodont.*, **7**, 516.

13. Stevens, A.J. (1980). A comparison of the effectiveness of variable diameter vs. unwaxed floss. *J. Periodontol.*, **51**, 666.

14. Bergenholtz, A., Bjorne, A. and Vikstrom, G. (1974). The plaque-removing ability of some common interdental aids. *J. Clin. Periodont.*, **1**, 160.

15. Brady, J.M., Gray, W.A. and Bhaskar, S.M. (1973). Electron microscopic study of the effect of water jet lavage devices on dental plaque. *J. Dent. Res.*, **52**, 1310.

16. Svatun, B., Saxton, C.A., Rolla, G. and van der Ouderaa, F. (1989). A 1-year study on the maintenance of gingival health by a dentifrice containing a zinc salt and non-anionic antimicrobial agent. *J. Clin. Periodont.*, **16**, 75.

17. Loe, H. and Rindom Schiot, C. (1970). The effect of mouthrinses and topical application of chlorhexidine on the development of dental plaque and gingivitis in man. *J. Periodont. Res.*, **5**, 79.

18. Pitcher, G.R., Newman, H.N. and Strahan, J.D. (1980). Access to subgingival plaque by disclosing agents using mouthrising and direct irrigation. *J. Clin. Periodont.*, **7**, 300.

19. Greenwell, H., Bakr, A., Bissada N., Debanne, S. and Rowland, D. (1985). The effect of Keyes' method of oral hygiene on the subgingival microflora compared to the effect of scaling and/or surgery. *J. Clin. Periodont.*, **12**, 327.

20. Walker, C.B. (1988). Microbiological effects of mouthrinses containing antimicrobials. *J. Clin. Periodont.*, **15**, 499.

21. Schroeder, H.E. and Scherle, W.F. (1988). Cemento-enamel junction—revisited. *J. Periodont. Res.*, **23**, 53.

22. Dowell, P. and Addy, M. (1983). Dentine hypersensitivity—A review: I Aetiology, symptoms and theories of pain production. *J. Clin. Periodont.*, **10**, 314.

23. Clark, D.C., Hanley, J.A., Geoghegan, S. and Vinet, D. (1985). The effectiveness of fluoride varnish and desensitizing toothpaste in treating dentinal hypersensitivity. *J. Periodont. Res.*, **20**, 212.

24. Addy, M. and Newcombe, R. (1987). Dentine hypersensitivity: a comparison of five toothpastes used during a 6-week treatment period. *Br. Dent. J.*, **163**, 45.

CHAPTER 10

1. Rabbani, G.M., Ash, M. and Caffese, R.G. (1981). The effectiveness of subgingival scaling and root planing in calculus removal. *J. Periodontol.*, **52**, 119.

2. Badersten, A., Nilveus, R. and Egelberg, J. (1981). Effect of nonsurgical periodontal therapy. I. Moderately advanced periodontitis. *J. Clin. Periodont.*, **8**, 57.

3. Lindhe, J., Nyman S. and Karring, T. (1982). Scaling and root planing in shallow pockets. *J. Clin. Periodont.*, **9**, 415.

4. Jones, S.J., Lozdan, J. and Boyde, A. (1972). Tooth surfaces treated in situ with periodontal instruments. *Br. Dent. J.*, **132**, 57.

5. Lie, T. and Meyer, K. (1977). Calculus removal and loss of tooth substance in response to different periodontal instruments. *J. Clin. Periodont.*, **4**, 250.

6. Thornton, S. and Garnick, J. (1982). Comparison of ultrasonic to hand instruments in the removal of subgingival plaque. *J. Periodontol.*, **53**, 35.

7. Suppipat, N. (1974). Ultrasonics in periodontics. *J. Clin. Periodont.*, **1**, 206.

8. Clark, S.M. (1969). The ultrasonic dental unit: A guide for clinical application of ultrasonics. *J. Periodontol.*, **40**, 621.

9. Holbrook, W.P., Muir, K.F., MacPhee, I.T. and Ross, P.W. (1978). Bacteriological investigation of the aerosol from ultrasonic scalers. *Br. Dent. J.*, **144**, 245.

10. Muir, K.F., Ross, P.W., MacPhee, I.T., Holbrook, W.P. and Kowolik, M.J. (1978). Reduction of microbial contamination from ultrasonic scalers. *Br. Dent. J.*, **145**, 76.

11. Walmsley, A.D., Walsh, T.F. and Laird, W.R.E. (1988). Ultrasonic instruments in dentistry. *Dental Update*, **15**, 321.

12. Lie, T. and Leknes, K.N. (1985). Evaluation of the effect on root surfaces of air turbine scalers and ultrasonic instrumentation. *J. Periodontol.*, **56**, 522.

13. Hatfield, C.G. and Baumhammers, A. (1971). Cytotoxic effects of periodontally involved surfaces of human teeth. *Arch. Oral Biol.*, **16**, 465.

14. Daly, C.G., Kieser, J.B., Corbet, E.F. and Seymour, G.J. (1979). Cementum involved in periodontal disease. A review of its features and clinical management. *J. Dent.*, **7**, 3.

15. Everhart, D.L., Dahab, O., Wolff, L. and Stahl, S.S. (1982). The further localization of antibody on cemental tissue. *J. Periodontol.*, **53**, 168.

16. Koichi, T., Hindman, R.E., O'Leary, T.J. and Kafrawy, A.H. (1985). Determination of the presence of root-bound endotoxin using the local Shwartzman phenomenon. *J. Periodontol.*, **56**, 8.

17. Adriaens, P.A., de Boever, J.A. and Loesche, W.J. (1988). Bacterial invasion in root cementum and radicular dentin of periodontally diseased teeth in humans. *J. Periodontol.*, **59**, 222.

18. Jones, W.A. and O'Leary, T.J. (1978). The effectiveness of in vivo root planing in removing bacterial endotoxin from the roots of periodontally involved teeth. *J. Periodontol.*, **49**, 337.

19. Sarbinoff, J.A., O'Leary, T.J. and Miller, C.H. (1983). The comparative effectiveness of various agents in detoxifying diseased root surfaces. *J. Periodontol.*, **54**, 77.

20. Moore, J., Wilson, M. and Kieser, J.B. (1986). The distribution of bacterial lipopolysaccharide (endotoxin) in relation to periodontally involved root surfaces. *J. Clin. Periodont.*, **13**, 748.

21. Assad, D.A., Dunlap, R.M., Weinberg, S.R. and Ahl, D.R. (1987). Biologic preparation of diseased root surfaces. An in vitro study. *J. Periodontol.*, **58**, 30.

22. Tal, H., Panno, J.M. and Vaidyanathan, T.K. (1985). Scanning electron microscope evaluation of wear of dental curettes during standardized root planing. *J. Periodontol.*, **56**, 532.

23. Paquette, O.E. and Levin, M.P. (1977). The sharpening of scaling instruments: I. An examination of principles. *J. Periodontol.*, **48**, 163.

24. Paquette, O.E. and Levin, M.P. (1977). The sharpening of scaling instruments: II. A preferred technique. *J. Periodontol.*, **48**, 169.

25. Lubow, R.M., Mayhew, R.B., Murray, G.H., Summitt, J.B. and Usseglio, R.J. (1984). The effects of two sharpening methods on the strength of a periodontal scaling instrument. *J. Periodontol.*, **55**, 410.

26. Zampa, S.T. and Green, E. (1972). Effect of polishing agents on root roughness. *J. Periodontol.*, **43**, 125.

27. Boyd, A. (1984). Airpolishing effects on enamel, dentine, cement and bone. *Br. Dent. J.*, **156**, 287.

28. Patterson, C.J.W. and McLundie, A.C. (1984). A comparison of the effects of two different prophylaxis regimes in vitro on some restorative dental materials. *Br. Dent. J.*, **157**, 166.

29. Polson, A.M., Kantor, M.E. and Zander H.A. (1979). Periodontal repair after reduction of inflammation. *J. Periodont. Res.*, **14**, 520.

CHAPTER 11

1. Waite, I.M. (1975). The present status of the gingivectomy procedure. *J. Clin. Periodont.*, **2**, 241.

2. Hecht, A. and App, G.R. (1974). Blood volume lost during gingivectomy using two different anaesthetic techniques. *J. Periodontol.*, **45**, 9.

3. Goldman, H.M. (1951). Gingivectomy. *Oral Sur., Oral Med., and Oral Path.* **4**, 1136.

CHAPTER 12

1. Waite, I.M. and Strahan, J.D. (1987). *A Colour Atlas of Periodontal Surgery*. Wolfe Medical Publications Ltd. London.

2. Friedman, N. (1962). Mucogingival surgery: the apically repositioned flap. *J. Periodontol.*, **33**, 328.

3. Johnson, R.H. (1976). Basic flap management. *Dent Clin. N. Am.*, **20**, 3.

CHAPTER 13

1. Polson, A.M., Kantor, M.E. and Zander, H.A. (1979). Periodontal repair after reduction of inflammation. *J. Periodont. Res.*, **14**, 520.

2. Miyasato, M.C. (1975). The periodontal abscess. *Periodontal Abstracts*, **23**, 53.

3. Kareha, M.J., Rosenberg, E.S. and Dehaven, H. (1981). Therapeutic considerations in the management of a periodontal abscess with an intrabony defect. *J. Clin. Periodont.*, **8**, 374.

4. Ellegaard, B. and Loe, H. (1971). New attachment of periodontal tissue after treatment of intrabony lesions. *J. Periodontol.*, **42**, 648.

5. Caton, J. and Zander, H.A. (1976). Osseous repair of an infrabony pocket without new attachment of connective tissue. *J. Clin. Periodont.*, **3**, 54.

6. Karring, T., Nyman, S. and Lindhe, J. (1980). Healing following implantation of periodontitis affected roots into bone tissue. *J. Clin. Periodont.*, **7**, 96.

7. Nyman, S., Gottlow, J., Karring, T. and Lindhe, J. (1982). The regenerative potential of the periodontal ligament. An experimental study in the monkey. *J. Clin. Periodont.*, **9**, 257.

8. Magnusson, I., Runstad, L., Nyman, S. and Lindhe, J. (1983). A long junctional epithelium — A locus minoris resistentiae in plaque infection. *J. Clin. Periodont.*, **10**, 333.

9. Beaumont, R.H., O'Leary, T.J. and Kafrawy, A.H. (1984). Relative resistance of long junctional epithelial adhesions and connective tissue attachments to plaque-induced inflammation. *J. Periodontol.*, **55**, 213.

10. Donnenfeld, O.W., Hoag, P.M. and Weissman, D.P. (1970). A clinical study of the effects of osteoplasty. *J. Periodontol.*, **41**, 131.

11. Wood, D.L., Hoag, P.M., Donnenfeld, O.W. and Rosenfeld, L.D. (1972). Alveolar crest reduction following full and partial thickness flaps. *J. Periodontol.*, **43**, 141.

12. Froum, S.J., Ortiz, M., Witkin, R.T., Thaler, R., Scopp, I.W. and Stahl, S.S. (1976). Osseous autografts. III. Comparison of osseous coagulum-bone blend implants with open curettage. *J. Periodontol.*, **47**, 287.

13. Evian, C.I., Rosenberg, E.S., Coslet, J.G. and Corn, H. (1982). The osteogenic activity of bone removed from healing extraction sockets in humans. *J. Periodontol.*, **53**, 81.

14. Schallhorn, R.G. (1972). Postoperative problem associated with iliac transplants. *J. Periodontol.*, **43**, 3.

15. Pearson, G.E., Rosen, S. and Deporter, D.A. (1981). Preliminary observations on the usefulness of a decalcified, freeze-dried cancellous bone allograft

material in periodontal surgery. *J. Periodontol., 2,* 55.

16. Waite, I.M., Galgut, P.M., Doyle, C. and Smith, R. (1987). The role of clinical implant materials in the surgical treatment of chronic periodontitis. *Clinical Materials, 2,* 293.

17. Froum, S.J., Kushner, L., Scopp, I.W. and Stahl, S.S. (1982). Case reports. Human clinical and histologic responses to Durapatite implants in intraosseous lesions. *J. Periodontol., 53,* 719.

18. Yukna, R.A., Mayer, E.T. and Brite, D.V. (1984). Longitudinal evaluation of Durapatite ceramic as an alloplastic implant in periodontal osseous defects after 3 years. *J. Periodontol., 55,* 633.

19. Baldock, W.T., Hutchens, L.H., McFall, W.T. and Simpson, D.M. (1985). An evaluation of tricalcium phosphate implants in human periodontal osseous defects in two patients. *J. Periodontol., 56,* 1.

20. Gottlow, J., Nyman, S., Lindhe, J., Karring, T. and Wennstrom, J. (1986). New attachment formation in the human periodontium by guided tissue regeneration. Case reports. *J. Clin. Periodont., 13,* 604.

21. Pontoriero, R. Nyman, S., Lindhe, J., Rosenberg, E. and Sanavi, F. (1987). Guided tissue regeneration in the treatment of furcation defects in man. *J. Clin. Periodont., 14,* 618.

22. Becker, W., Becker, B.E., Prichard, J.F., Caffesse, R., Rosenberg, E. and Gian-Grasso, J. (1987). Root isolation for new attachment procedures — a surgical and suturing method. *J. Periodontol., 58,* 819.

23. Magnusson, I., Batich, C. and Collins, B.R. (1988). New attachment formation following controlled tissue regeneration using biodegradable membranes. *J. Periodontol., 59,* 1.

24. Egelberg, J., (1987). Regeneration and repair of periodontal tissues. *J. Periodont., Res., 22,* 233.

CHAPTER 14

1. Simon, J.H.S., Glik, D.H. and Frank, A.L. (1972). The relationship of endodontic-periodontic lesions. *J. Periodontol., 43,* 202.

2. Hildebrand, C.N. and Morse, D.R. (1980). Periodontic-endodontic interrelationships. *Dent. Clin. N. Am., 24,* 797.

3. Gold, S.I. and Moskow, B.S. (1987). Periodontal repair of periapical lesions: the borderland between pulpal and periodontal disease. *J. Clin. Periodont., 14,* 251.

4. Larato, D.C. (1970). Furcation involvements. Incidence and distribution. *J. Periodontol., 41,* 499.

5. Dunlap, R.M. and Gher, M.E. (1985). Root surface measurements of the mandibular first molar. *J. Periodontol., 56,* 234.

6. Hou, G.I. and Tsai, C.C. (1987). Relationship between periodontal furcation involvement and molar cervical enamel projections. *J. Periodontol., 58,* 715.

7. Tarnow, D. and Fletcher, P. (1984). Classification of the vertical component of furcation involvement. *J. Periodontol., 55,* 283.

8. Kalkwarf, K.L. and Reinhardt, R.A. (1988). The furcation problem: current controversies and future directions. *Dent. Clin. N. Am., 32,* 243.

9. Ross, I.F. and Thompson, R.H. (1978). A long term study of root retention in the treatment of maxillary molars with furcation involvement. *J. Periodontol., 49,* 238.

10. Bjorn, A.-L. and Hjort, P. (1982). Bone loss of furcated mandibular molars. A longitudinal study. *J. Clin. Periodont., 9,* 402.

11. Klinge, B., Nilveus, R., Kiger, R.D. and Egelberg, J. (1981). Effect of flap placement and defect size on healing of experimental furcation defects. *J. Periodontol., 16,* 236.

12. Pontoriero, R., Nyman, S., Lindhe, J., Rosenberg, E. and Sanavi, F. (1987). Guided tissue regeneration in the treatment of furcation defects in man. *J. Clin. Periodont., 14,* 618.

13. Hamp, S.F., Nyman, S. and Lindhe, J. (1975). Periodontal treatment of multirooted teeth. Results after 5 years. *J. Clin. Periodont., 2,* 126.

14. Langer, B., Stein, S.D. and Wagenberg, B. (1981). An evaluation of root resections — a ten-year study. *J. Periodontol., 12,* 719.

15. Erpenstein, H. (1983). A 3-year study of hemisectioned molars. *J. Clin. Periodont.*, **10**, 1.

16. Kalkwarf, K.L. and Reinhardt, R.A. (1988). The furcation problem: current controversies and future directions. *Dent. Clin. N. Am.*, **32**, 243.

17. Bower, R.C. (1979) Furcation morphology relative to periodontal treatment — furcation entrance architecture. *J. Periodontol.*, **50**, 23.

18. Bower, R.C. (1979) Furcation morphology relative to periodontal treatment — furcation root surface anatomy. *J. Periodontol.*, **50**, 336.

19. Newell, D.H. (1981). Current status of the management of teeth with furcation invasions. *J. Periodontol.*, **52**, 559.

20. Leon, L.E. and Vogel, R.I. (1987). A comparison of the effectiveness of hand scaling and ultrasonic debridement in furcations as evaluated by differential dark-field microscopy. *J. Periodontol.*, **57**, 86.

21. Appleton, I.E. (1980). Restoration of root-resected teeth. *J. Prosth. Dent.*, **44**, 150.

22. Hermann, D.W., Gher, M.E., Dunlap, R.M. and Pelleu, G.B. (1983). The potential attachment area of the maxillary first molar. *J. Periodontol.*, **54**, 431.

CHAPTER 15

1. Bowers, G.M. (1963). A study of the width of attached gingiva. *J. Periodontol.*, **34**, 201.

2. Baker, D.L. and Seymour, G.J. (1976). The possible pathogenesis of gingival recession. A histological study of induced recession in the rat. *J. Clin. Periodont.*, **3**, 208.

3. Hall, W.B. (1981). The current status of mucogingival problems and their therapy. *J. Periodontol.*, **52**, 569.

4. Miller, P.D. (1988). Regenerative and reconstructive periodontic plastic surgery. *Dent. Clin. N. Am.*, **32**, 287.

5. Lang, N.P. and Loe, H. (1972). The relationship between width of keratinized gingiva and gingival health. *J. Periodontol.*, **43**, 623.

6. Miyasato, M., Crigger, M. and Egelberg, J. (1977). Gingival condition in areas of minimal and appreciable width of keratinized gingiva. *J. Clin. Periodont.*, **4**, 200.

7. Wennstrom, J. and Lindhe, J. (1983). Role of attached gingiva for maintenance of periodontal health. *J. Clin. Periodont.*, **10**, 206.

8. Kisch, J., Badersten, A. and Egelberg, J. (1986). Longitudinal observation of 'unattached', mobile gingival areas. *J. Clin. Periodont.*, **13**, 131.

9. Ericsson, I. and Lindhe, J. (1984). Recession in sites with inadequate width of the keratinized gingiva. An experimental study in the dog. *J. Clin. Periodont.*, **11**, 95.

10. Kennedy, J.E., Bird, W.C., Palcanis, K.G. and Dorfman, H.S. (1985). A longitudinal evaluation of varying widths of attached gingiva. *J. Clin. Periodont.*, **12**, 667.

11. Stetler, K.J. and Bissada, N.F. (1987). Significance of the width of keratinized gingiva on the periodontal status of teeth with submarginal restorations. *J. Periodontol.*, **58**, 696.

12. Ferguson, M.W. and Rix, C. (1983). Pathogenesis of abnormal midline spacing of human central incisors. *Br. Dent. J.*, **154**, 212.

13. Matter, J. (1982). Free gingival grafts for the treatment of gingival recession. A review of some techniques. *J. Clin. Periodont.*, **9**, 103.

14. Heaney, T.G. (1974). A reappraisal of environment, function and gingival specificity. *J. Periodontol.*, **45**, 695.

15. Karring, T., Cumming, B.R., Oliver, R.C. and Loe, H. (1975). The origin of granulation tissue and its impact on postoperative results of mucogingival surgery. *J. Periodontol.*, **46**, 577.

16. Dordick, B., Coslet, J.G. and Seibert, J.S. (1976). I. Clinical evaluation of free autogenous gingival grafts placed on alveolar bone. II. Coverage of non-pathologic dehiscences and fenestration. *J. Periodontol.*, **47**, 559 and 568.

17. Caffesse, R.G., Burgett, F.G. Nasjleti, C.E. and Castelli, W.A. (1979). Healing of free gingival grafts with and without periosteum. I. Histologic evaluation. *J. Periodontol.*, **50**, 586.

18. Busshop, J., de Boever, J. and Schautteet, H. (1983). Revascularization of gingival autografts placed on different receptor beds. A fluoroangiographic study. *J. Clin. Periodont.*, **10**, 327.

19. Sullivan, H.C. and Atkins, J.H. (1968). Free autogenous gingival grafts: principles of successful grafting. *Periodontics*, **6**, 21.

20. Ward, V.J. (1974). A clinical assessment of the use of the free gingival graft for correcting localized recession associated with frenal pull. *J. Periodontol.*, **45**, 78.

21. Hangorsky, U. and Bissada, N.F. (1980). Clinical assessment of free gingival graft effectiveness on the maintenance of periodontal health. *J. Periodontol.*, **51**, 5.

22. Dorfman, H.S., Kennedy, J.E. and Bird, W.C. (1982). Longitudinal evaluation of free autogenous gingival grafts — a four year report. *J. Periodontol.*, **53**, 349.

23. Allen, E.P. (1988). Use of mucogingival procedures to enhance esthetics *Dent. Clin. N. Am.*, **32**, 307.

24. Edel, A. (1974). Clinical evaluation of free connective tissue grafts used to increase the width of keratinised gingiva. *J. Clin. Periodont.*, **1**, 185.

25. Douglas, G.L. (1976). Mucogingival repairs in periodontal surgery. *Dent. Clin. N. Am.*, **20**, 107.

26. de Waal, H., Kon, S. and Ruben, M.P. (1988). The laterally positioned flap. *Dent. Clin. N. Am.*, **32**, 267.

27. Waite, I.M. (1984). An assessment of the postsurgical results following the combined laterally positioned flap and gingival graft procedure. *Quintessence International Dental Digest*, **4**, 441.

28. Sugarman, E.F. (1969). A clinical and histological study of the attachment of grafted tissue to bone and teeth. *J. Periodontol.*, **40**, 381.

29. Cohen, D.W. and Ross, S.E. (1968). The double papillae repositioned flap in periodontal therapy. *J. Periodontol.*, **39**, 65.

30. Bernimoulin, J.P., Luscher, B. and Muhlemann, H.R. (1975). Coronally repositioned periodontal flap. *J. Clin. Periodont.*, **2**, 1.

31. Caffesse, R.G. and Guinard, E.A. (1978). Treatment of localised gingival recessions, II. Coronally repositioned flap with a free gingival graft. *J. Periodontol.*, **49**, 357.

CHAPTER 16

1. Wentz, F.M., Jarabak, J. and Orban, B. (1958). Experimental occlusal trauma imitating cuspal interference. *J. Periodont.*, **29**, 117.

2. Svanberg, G. and Lindhe, J. (1974). Vascular reactions in the periodontal ligament incident to trauma from occlusion. *J. Clin. Periodont.*, **1**, 58.

3. Meitner, S.A. (1975). Codestructive factors of marginal periodontitis and repetitive mechanical injury. *J. Dent. Res.*, **54**, Special issue C, 78.

4. Polson, A.M. (1980). Inter-relationship of inflammation and tooth mobility (trauma) in pathogenesis of periodontal disease. *J. Clin. Periodont.*, **7**, 351.

5. Perrier, M. and Polson, A. (1982). The effect of progressive and increasing tooth hypermobility on reduced but healthy periodontal supporting tissues. *J. Periodontol.*, **53**, 152.

6. Nyman, S. and Lindhe, J. (1977). Consideration on the design of occlusion in prosthetic rehabilitation of patients with advanced periodontal disease. *J. Clin. Periodont.*, **4**, 1.

7. Bernstein, M. (1969). Orthodontics in periodontal and prosthetic therapy. *J. Periodontol.*, **40**, 577.

8. Behlfelt, K., Ericsson, L., Jacobson, L. and Linder-Aronson, S. (1981). The occurrence of plaque and gingivitis and its relationship to tooth alignment within the dental arches. *J. Clin. Periodont.*, **8**, 329.

9. Griffiths, G.S. and Addy, M. (1981). Effects of malalignment of teeth in the anterior segments on plaque accumulation. *J. Clin. Periodont.*, **8**, 481.

10. Ainamo, J. (1972). Relationship between malalignment of teeth and periodontal disease. *Scand. J. Dent. Res.*, **80**, 104.

11. Zachrisson, S. and Zachrisson, B.W. (1972). Gingival condition associated with orthodontic treatment. *Angle Orthodont.*, **42**, 26.

12. Zachrisson, B.W. and Alnaes, L. (1973). Periodontal condition in orthodontically treated and untreated individuals I. *Angle Orthodont.*, **43**, 402.

13. Zachrisson, B.W. and Alnaes, L. (1974). Periodontal condition in orthodontically treated and untreated individuals II. *Angle Orthodont.*, **44**, 48.

14. Lundstrom, F., Hamp, S. and Nyman, S. (1980). Systematic plaque control in children undergoing long-term orthodontic treatment. *European J. Orthodont.*, **2**, 27.

15. Buckley, L.A. (1981). The relationships between malocclusion, gingival inflammation, plaque and calculus. *J. Periodontol.*, **52**, 35.

16. Poulton, D.R. and Aaronson, S.A. (1961). The relationship between occlusion and periodontal status. *Am. J. Orthodont.*, **47**, 690.

17. Wise, M.D. (1986). *Occlusion and restorative dentistry for the general practitioner.* British Dental Association. London.

18. Dawson, P.E. (1974). *Occlusal problems.* C.V. Mosby Co. St. Louis.

CHAPTER 17

1. Leon, A.R. (1977). The periodontium and restorative procedures. *J. Oral Rehab.*, **4**, 105.

2. Gorzo, I., Newman, H.N. and Strahan, J.D. (1979). Amalgam restorations, plaque removal and periodontal health. *J. Clin. Periodont.*, **6**, 98.

3. Hall, W.B. (1980). Periodontal preparation of the mouth for restoration. *Dent. Clin. N. Am.,* **24**, 195.

4. Ingber, J.S. (1976). Forced eruption: part II. A method of treating nonrestorable teeth — periodontal and restorative considerations. *J. Periodontol.*, **47**, 203.

5. Perrier, M. and Polson, A. (1982). The effect of progressive and increasing tooth hypermobility on reduced but healthy periodontal supporting tissues. *J. Periodontol.*, **53**, 152.

6. Vale, J.D.F. and Caffesse, R.G. (1979). Removal of amalgam overhangs — a profilometric and scanning electron microscope evaluation. *J. Periodontol.*, **50**, 245.

7. Spinks, G.C, Carson, R.E., Hancock, E.B. and Pelleu, G.B. (1986). An SEM study of overhang removal methods. *J. Periodontol.*, **57**, 632.

8. Wise, M.D. (1985). Stability of gingival crest after surgery and before anterior crown replacement. *J. Prosth. Dent.*, **53**, 20.

9. Bergman, B., Hugoson, A. and Olsson, C. (1977). Caries and periodontal status in patients fitted with removable dentures. *J. Clin. Periodont.*, **4**, 134.

10. Bates, J.F. and Addy, M. (1978). Partial dentures and plaque accumulation. *J. Dent.*, **4**, 285.

11. Ghamrawy, el, E. (1979). Qualitative changes in dental plaque formation related to removable partial dentures. *J. Oral Rehabil.*, **6**, 183.

12. Hobkirk, J.A. and Strahan, J.D. (1979). The influence on the gingival tissues of prostheses incorporating gingival relief area. *J. Dent.*, **17**, 15.

13. Rantanen, T., Siirila, H.S. and Lehvila, P. (1980). Effect of instruction and motivation on dental knowledge and behaviour among wearers of partial dentures. *Acta. Odontol. Scand.*, **38**, 9.

14. Nyman, S., Lindhe, J. and Lundgren, D. (1975). The role of occlusion for the stability of fixed bridges in patients with reduced periodontal tissue support. *J. Clin. Periodont.*, **2**, 53.

15. Nyman, S. and Lindhe, J. (1979). A longitudinal study of combined periodontal and prosthetic treatment of patients with advanced periodontal disease. *J. Periodontol.*, **50**, 163.

16. Potashnick, S.R. and Rosenberg, E.S. (1982). Forced eruption principles in periodontal and restorative dentistry. *J. Prosth. Dent.*, **48**, 141.

APPENDIX 3

1. Loe, H. and Silness, J. (1963). Periodontal disease in pregnancy. *Acta. Odontol. Scand.*, **21**, 533.

2. Silness, J. and Loe, H. (1964). Periodontol disease in pregnancy. II. *Acta. Odontol. Scand.*, **22**, 121.

3. Russell, A.L. (1956). A system of classification and scoring for prevalence surveys of periodontal disease. *J. Dent. Res.*, **36**, 922.

4. Ramfjord, S.P. (1959). Indices for prevalence and incidence of periodontal disease. *J. Periodontol.*, **30**, 51.

5. Ainamo, J., Barnes, D., Beagrie, G., Cutress, T., Martin, J. and Sardo Infirri, J. (1988). Development of the World Health Organization Community Periodontal Index of Treatment Needs. *Int. Dent. J.*, **32**, 281.

6. Greene, J.C. and Vermillion, J.R. (1960). Oral Hygiene Index: a method for classifying oral hygiene status. *J. Am. Dent. Assoc.*, **61**, 172.

7. Loe, H. (1967). The Gingival Index, the Plaque Index and the Retention Index systems. *J. Periodontol.*, **38**, Supplement, 610.

8. Muhlemann, H.R. (1976). Psychological and chemical mediators of gingival health. *Journal of Preventative Dentistry*, **4**, 6.

9. O'Leary, T.J., Drake, R.B. and Naylor, J.E. (1972). The Plaque Control Record. *J. Periodontol.*, **43**, 38.

10. Miller, S.C. (1950). *Textbook of Periodontia*. The Blakeston Co. Philadelphia.

11. Grant, D.A., Stern, I.B. and Listgarten, M.A. (1988). *Periodontics, Sixth Edition*. C.V. Mosby Co. St. Louis.

APPENDIX 6

1. Daly, C.G., Kieser, J.B., Corbet, E.F. and Seymour, G.J. (1979). Cementum involved in periodontal disease. A review of its features and clinical management. *J. Dent.*, **7**, 3.

2. Wirthlin, M.R. and Hancock, E.B. (1980). Biologic preparation of diseased root surfaces. *J. Periodontol.*, **51**, 291.

3. Wirthlin, M.R. and Hancock, E.B. (1981). Chemical treatment of diseased root surfaces in vitro. *J. Periodontol.*, **52**, 694.

4. Sarbinoff, J.A., O'Leary, T.J. and Miller, C.H. (1983). The comparative effectiveness of various agents in detoxifying diseased root surfaces. *J. Periodontol.*, **54**, 77.

5. Fernyhough, W. and Page, R.C. (1983). Attachment, growth and synthesis by human gingival fibroblasts on demineralised or fibronectin-treated normal and diseased tooth roots. *J. Periodontol.*, **54**, 133.

6. Daly, C.G. (1982). Anti-bacterial effect of citric acid treatment of periodontally diseased root surfaces in vitro. *J. Clin. Periodont.*, **6**, 386.

7. Bogle, G., Crigger, M., Egelberg, J. and Garrett, S. (1983). New connective tissue attachment in beagles with advanced natural periodontitis. *J. Periodont. Res.*, **18**, 220.

8. Olson, R.H., Adams, D.F. and Layman, D.L. (1985). Inhibitory effect of periodontally diseased root extracts on the growth of human gingival fibroblasts. *J. Periodontol.*, **56**, 592.

9. Polson, A.M. and Proye, M.P. (1982). Effect of root surface alterations on periodontal healing. II. Citric acid treatment of the denuded root. *J. Clin. Periodont.*, **9**, 441.

10. Albair, W.B., Cobb, C.M. and Killoy W.J. (1982). Connective tissue attachment to periodontally diseased roots after citric acid demineralization. *J. Periodontol.*, **53**, 515.

11. Stahl, S.S. and Froum, S.J. (1977). Human clinical and histological repair responses following the use of citric acid in periodontal therapy. *J. Periodontol.*, **48**, 261.

12. Kashani H.G., Magner, A.W. and Stahl, S.S. (1984). The effect of root planing and citric acid applications on flap healing in humans. A histologic evaluation. *J. Periodontol.*, **55**, 679.

APPENDIX 7

1. Newcombe, G.M. and Waite, I.M. (1972). The effectiveness of two local analgesic preparations in reducing haemorrhage during periodontal surgery. *J. Dent.*, **1**, 37.

2. Hecht, A. and App, G.R. (1974). Blood volume lost during gingivectomy using two different anaesthetic techniques. *J. Periodontol.*, **45**, 9.

APPENDIX 8

1. Axelsson, P. and Lindhe, J. (1974). The effect of a preventive programme on dental plaque, gingivitis and caries in schoolchildren. Results after one and two years. *J. Clin Periodont.*, **1**, 126.

2. Axelsson, P. and Lindhe, J. (1981). The significance of maintenance care in the treatment of periodontal disease. *J. Clin. Periodont.*, **8**, 281.

3. Axelsson, P. and Lindhe, J. (1981). Effect of controlled oral hygiene procedures on caries and periodontal disease in adults. Results after 6 years. *J. Clin. Periodont.*, **8**, 239.

4. Badersten, A., Nilveus, R. and Egelberg, J. (1981). Effect of nonsurgical periodontal therapy. I. Moderately advanced periodontitis. *J. Clin. Periodont.* **8**, 57.

5. Badersten, A., Nilveus, R. and Egelberg, J. (1987). 4-year observations of basic periodontal therapy. *J. Clin. Periodont.*, **14**, 438.

6. Rabbani, G.M., Ash, M. and Caffese, R.G. (1981). The effectiveness of subgingival scaling and root planing in calculus removal. *J. Periodontol.*, **52**, 119.

7. Badersten, A., Nilveus, R. and Egelberg, J. (1985). Effect of nonsurgical periodontal therapy. VII. Bleeding, suppuration and probing depth in sites with probing attachment loss. *J. Clin. Periodont.*, **12**, 432.

8. Lindhe, J., Socransky, S.S., Nyman, S., Haffajee, A. and Westfelt, E. (1982). Critical probing depths in periodontal therapy. *J. Clin. Periodont.*, **9**, 323.

9. Lindhe, J., Westfelt, E., Nyman, S., Socransky, S.S., Heijl, L. and Bratthall, G. (1982). Healing following surgical/non-surgical treatment of periodontal disease. A clinical study. *J. Clin. Periodont.*, **9**, 115.

10. Ramfjord, S.P. (1987). Maintenance care for treated periodontitis patients. *J. Clin Periodont.*, **14**, 433.

11. Rosling, B., Nyman, S. and Lindhe, J. (1976). The effect of systematic plaque control on bone regeneration in infrabony pockets. *J. Clin. Periodont.*, **3**, 38.

12. Lindhe, J. and Nyman, S. (1984). Long-term maintenance of patients treated for advanced periodontal disease. *J. Clin. Periodont.*, **11**, 504.

13. Nyman, S., Rosling, B. and Lindhe, J. (1975). Effect of professional tooth cleaning on healing after periodontal surgery. *J. Clin. Periodont.*, **2**, 80.

14. Nyman, S., Lindhe, J. and Rosling, B. (1977). Periodontal surgery in plaque-infected dentitions. *J. Clin. Periodont.*, **4**, 240.

APPENDIX 9

1. Krejci, R.F., Kalkwarf, K.L. and Krause-Hohenstein, U. (1987). Electrosurgery — a biological approach. *J. Clin. Periodont.*, **14**, 557.

2. Azzi, R., Kenney, E.B., Tsao, T.F. and Carranza, F.A. (1983). The effect of electrosurgery on alveolar bone. *J. Periodontol.*, **54**, 96.

3. Hurt, W.C., Nabers, C.L. and Rose, G.G. (1972). Some clinical and histologic observations of gingiva treated by cryotherapy. *J. Periodontol.*, **43**, 151.

4. Severin, C. (1988). Carbon dioxide laser training course. *Br. Dent. J.*, **165**, 268.

5. Pick, R.M., Pecaro, B.C. and Silberman, C.J. (1985). The laser gingivectomy. The use of the CO_2 laser for the removal of phenytoin hyperplasia. *J. Periodontol.*, **56**, 492.

APPENDIX 12

1. American Academy of Periodontology (1986). Glossary of Periodontic Terms. *J. Periodontol.* Supplement.

2. Magnusson, I., Runstad, L., Nyman, S. and Lindhe, J. (1983). A long junctional epithelium—A locus minoris resistentiae in plaque infection. *J. Clin. Periodont.*, **10**, 333.

3. Levine, H.E. (1972). Periodontal flap surgery with gingival fiber retention. *J. Periodontol.*, **43**, 91.

4. Yukna, R.A. and Williams, J.E. (1980). Five year evaluation of the excisional new attachment procedure. *J. Periodontol.*, **51**, 382.

5. Dello Russo, N.M. (1981). Use of the fiber retention procedure in treating the maxillary anterior region. *J. Periodontol.*, **52**, 208.

6. Nyman, S., Gottlow, J., Karring, T. and Lindhe, J. (1982). The regenerative potential of the periodontal ligament. An experimental study in the monkey. *J. Clin. Periodont.*, **9**, 257.

7. Egelberg, J. (1987). Regeneration and repair of periodontal tissues. *J. Periodont. Res.*, **22**, 233.

8. Stahl, S.S., Slavkin, H.C., Yamada, L. and Levine, S. (1972). Speculations about gingival repair. *J. Periodontol.*, **43**, 395.

9. Donnenfeld, O.W., Marks, R. and Glickman, I. (1964). The apically respositioned flap. *J. Periodontol.*, **35**, 381.

10. Costitch, E.R. and Ramfjord, S.P. (1968). Healing after periosteal exposure. *J. Periodontol.*, **39**, 199.

11. Costitch, E.R. and Ramfjord, S.P. (1968). Healing after partial denudation of the alveolar process. *J. Periodontol.*, **39**, 127.

INDEX

All references are to page numbers

A

Abutment teeth, 123
Acid-etched bridge and splint, 129
Acquired immune deficiency syndrome (AIDS), 48, 54
Actinobacillus actinomycetemcomitans, 27, 29, 30
  periodontal abscess, 37
Actinomyces, 17, 18
Acute herpetic gingivo-stomatitis, 42-43
Acute monocytic leukaemia, 34
Acute necrotising ulcerative gingivitis, 25, 41
Acute periodontal conditions, 37-43
Aetiology of periodontal diseases, 17-19, 141
Agranulocytosis, 34
Alveolar mucosa, 12
Analgesia, local, 68, 77, 152
Antibiotics, 26, 28, 29, 30, 65
Aphthous ulcers, 47
Antiseptic mouthwash, 65, 66, 155
Arsenic, systemic, 36
Aspirin, causing lesion, 47
Assessment forms, 144-149

B

Bacterial irritants, control, 122
Bacteroides, 18, 19
Bacteroides forsythus, 19
Bacteroides intermedius, 19, 49
Bacteroides gingivalis, 19, 29, 30
Bacteroides melaninogenicus, 33
Basement lamina, 11
Benign mucous membrane pemphigoid, 33
Bismuth, systemic, 36
Blake knife, 79
Bleeding, on probing, 19, 59, 153
  index, 143
Blood dyscrasias, 34
Blood vessels, 9
B-lymphocytes, 21, 22, 141
Bone
  alveolar, 9, 10
  marginal, 10
Bone defects, 158-159
  treatment, 91-100
    acute lesion repair, 92
    after root planing and plaque control, 91-92
    chronic lesion repair, 93-94
    extraction of tooth/root, 91
    grafts, 95-96
    healing of defect, 94
    implants, 96-97
    new attachment, 91
    osseous surgery, 94-95
    regeneration, 91, 98-100
    repair, 91
Bone substitutes, 95
Bridges
  acid-etched, 129
  inadequate, 131
  treated teeth with loss of periodontal support, 136-137
Bruxism, 56

C

Calculus
  formation theories, 23
  subgingival, 23, 68, 69
    detection 69
  supragingival, 23
Cancrum oris (noma), 41
Cell migration, 98
Chalones, 98
Chemical injury, 97
Chemotactic factors, 22
Children
  pre-school, 49
  teenage, 50
Chisel scaler, 71
Chlorhexidine, 65-66
CPITN probe, 58
Citric acid, 151
Classification of periodontal disease, 140
Clenching, 56
Cohn plasma fraction IV, 151
Collagenase, 27
Congenital abnormalities, 15
Contact point, 13
Contaminated cementum, 75
  treatment, 151
Corium, 12
  elastic fibres, 12
Coronally repositioned gingival graft, 118-119
Crown margins, defective, 23
Cryosurgery, 157
Curettes, 74-75
Cyclosporin, 36

D

Dehiscences, 10
Dental floss, 63
  holder, 64
  superfloss, 64
  threaders, 64
Dental history, 54
Dentifrices, 65
  desensitising, 67
Desquamative gingivitis, 33, 48
Developmental abnormalities, 15
Diabetes mellitus, 33, 54
Disclosing agent, 60, 66
Double papillary flap, 118
Down's syndrome, 31
Drugs, 35-36, 54, 65

E

Electric tooth brush, 62
Electrosurgery, 157
Endodontic lesion, primary, 38, 101
  combined endodontic/periodontal lesion, 102
  with secondary periodontal involvement, 101-102
Endodontics, surgical, with periodontal surgery, 134-135
Endotoxin, 20, 22
Enzymes, 18, 20, 27, 141